POSTVIRAL
FATIGUE SYNDROME

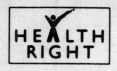

**HEALTH
RIGHT**

POSTVIRAL
FATIGUE SYNDROME

Its Causes and How to Heal It

LEON CHAITOW

JM Dent & Sons Ltd
London

First published 1989
© Leon Chaitow 1989

This book is set in 10½ on 12½pt Palatino by
Deltatype Ltd, Ellesmere Port, Cheshire
Printed in Great Britain by
Guernsey Press Co. Ltd, Guernsey, C.I. for
J. M. Dent & Sons Ltd
91 Clapham High Street, London SW4 7TA

British Library Cataloguing in Publication Data

Chaitow, Leon
    Postviral fatigue Syndrome
    1.Man.Myalgic encephalomyelitis
    I.Title II.Series
    616.8'3

    ISBN 0-460-12593-1

Contents

Acknowledgments   vi

THE CAUSES OF ME

1 What Is ME?   3
2 The Virus Connection: Cause or Consequence?   15
3 The Mind, the Immune System and ME   31
4 Hyperventilation and ME   42
5 Allergy, Toxicity and ME   47
6 The Candida-ME Link   61
7 Nutrition as Immune Enhancer and Immune
  Suppressor   72
8 ME, Sleep, Exercise, Environment and Lifestyle   89

THE HEALING OF ME

9 Dietary and Supplementation Strategies   101
10 Harnessing Mind Power   129
11 Antiviral Methods   154
12 Additional Healing Methods for ME   171
13 Current Medical Thinking and ME   182

List of Resources   190
Index   195

Acknowledgments

ME was brought into focus for me by Sue Finlay who referred to my book on candida albicans as having helped her towards enhanced recovery, in her article in the *Observer* ('An Illness Doctors Don't Recognise', 1 June 1986). I contacted Sue and we became correspondents, exchanging information and ideas. I realized through the knowledge and information which was opened up for me by Sue that I had been treating ME for some time, without being aware of the fact.

I had long been dealing with candida overgrowth, nutritional deficiencies, food sensitivities and allergies, heavy metal toxicities, hyperventilation and stress-related anxieties and depression. Chronic fatigue was a feature of many of these conditions and in some was the main symptom. I had of course heard of Royal Free disease and had read of postviral fatigue syndrome. What I had not done was to see the interconnection which all too often exists between these different conditions when they all meet at the focal point of the body's defences, the immune system.

Toxicity, stress and deficiency as well as persistent yeast

overgrowth and allergy all deplete and exhaust the immune system. So, of course, does subsequent and persistent viral activity which can result from this weakened state of our defences.

Hyperventilation, exhaustion and depression are natural outcomes of such conditions and make matters worse. A cycle can ensue in which the interaction of causes and symptoms becomes blurred. In deciding where to make a therapeutic intervention a complex hunt for the chicken and the egg becomes apparent. Do we start with stress-reduction and breathing retraining or with nutritional supplementation or immune enhancement or by attacking the persistent yeast overgrowth or viral activity?

ME was the link for me and it arrived just as I was becoming increasingly involved in, and aware of, the ways in which AIDS also contained these elements, but of course in much greater degree. The revelation that some people with AIDS were turning their conditions around and were using a variety of holistic, orthodox and alternative, methods to do so coincided with my awareness that this was also the way in which the complicated fatigue, burn-out, conditions which I was treating should be handled (whether viral connections could be established or not). Only by dealing with the mind/body unit comprehensively, providing for all of its needs, could the homoeostatic, self-healing mechanisms begin to operate to restore health.

For this knowledge I am indebted to all of my patients who have taught me so much, and to the many people who have shared knowledge with me over the past years, too many in fact to list for I would certainly forget someone. So I give acknowledgment to, and dedicate this book to, all those with fatigue, postviral or otherwise, and to Sue Finlay in particular. This remarkable woman has throughout her recovery, and even when in the worst extremes of exhaustion, continued to educate, share knowledge,

Acknowledgments

badger officialdom and the medical powers-that-be, seek answers and maintain tirelessly (not true, she was tired but you understand what I mean) her determination to see ME dealt with properly in our society, by the government, the media, the medical profession and the public at large. She has nearly won her battle, I believe, although talk of 'yuppie flu' must be almost enough to set her screaming.

Thank you Sue.

Part I

THE CAUSES OF ME

1 What Is ME?

What's in a Name?

A look at the various names which have been given to this condition over the years teaches a great deal about its history and also much about the way it has been viewed by the medical opinion of the moment.

A major outbreak of this mysterious condition occurred in Los Angeles in 1934 where almost 5 per cent of the nursing and medical staff at major hospitals were affected. Over half of these were still ill after six months. In Iceland in 1948 around 500 people suddenly became ill with the symptoms of acute ME in what came to be called Icelandic disease, and over half were still ill when re-examined seven years later. In London in 1955 almost 300 of the staff (and a few patients) at the Royal Free Hospital were struck down with the illness, thus giving it a name still commonly used, Royal Free disease.

It was a study of this last outbreak by two physicians Drs McEvedy and Beard in 1970 which labelled the condition as having 'hysterical' origins, in contrast to the opinions of many of the doctors who had been affected – some for a period of years – when working at the Royal Free, who were convinced that their illness had physical origins. Regrettably this somewhat judgmental term 'mass hysteria', with its suggestions of fakery, neurosis and imitated behaviour, has acted as a barrier to the recognition that at least some of the background to ME relates, in many if not all instances, to immune suppression resulting from mental and emotional factors.

Some of the other terms used to describe ME (myalgic encephalomyelitis) include 'epidemic neuromyasthenia', 'benign myalgic encephalomyelitis', 'yuppie flu', 'closet AIDS', 'chronic Epstein-Barr virus syndrome' and 'chronic mononucleosis-like syndrome'.

These latter terms, including 'closet AIDS', recognize that, in some instances at least, a viral infection is either a predisposing or a continuing element of the condition. This recognition usually fails, though, to look at why the individual thus affected was so susceptible to a common viral activity in the first place, and why the complaint became chronic rather than being swiftly dealt with by the immune system.

Australian researchers have examined 200 people with this condition and have come to the conclusion, shared by the US Center of Disease Control, that it should be called chronic fatigue syndrome (CFS). They argue that many patients have no myalgic or encephalitis history; they also argue (correctly) that the viral connection is not present in all people with the syndrome, and therefore that 'postviral' is an inappropriate term. They suggest that because ME has a connotation of hysteria, a clearly invalid hypothesis they believe, the ultimate term should be CFS until a clearer pathophysiology is defined.

The popular term current in the UK, however, remains 'postviral fatigue syndrome', which seems reasonable in those instances where viral activity can be shown to have

4

precipitated the condition. Attempts in the UK and USA to find a single causative agent have failed, since plainly no single infecting agent is involved. Rather, there are a multitude of possible culprits and, in addition and more importantly, the 'susceptibility factor'.

The really central question in the end is what allows one agent or another to produce the symptoms of ME in one person and not in another. The cause of a condition such as this must lie in that answer, whether it be immune depression due to toxicity, deficiency, allergy, emotional factors, recurrent infection or, as seems likely, a combination of such 'causes'. If ME is a sort of 'mini' or 'closet' AIDS, without that condition's darker implications, we come to understand that many causes lead to it and a variety of helpful immune-supporting avenues exist to aid recovery.

The term myalgic encephalomyelitis (ME) does not define its causes but rather its major symptoms and this then would seem to be the current term of choice, and the one which I shall use throughout this book.

Symptoms of ME

The main symptoms found in people diagnosed as having myalgic encephalomyelitis (ME), often called postviral fatigue syndrome (PVFS), are listed below. They are:

- Chronic fatigue.
- Extreme fatiguability of muscles (they tire very quickly indeed).
- Aching muscles and/or joints.
- Low-grade fever.
- Headache.
- Inability to concentrate and poor memory ('woolly brain syndrome').

- Swollen lymph glands.
- Very cold extremities.
- Sleep disturbances.
- Sore throat.
- Gastro-intestinal discomfort.
- Depression and emotional distress (anxiety, panic attacks).
- Dizziness, palpitations, numb and tingling limbs.
- A variety of disturbances of organs of sense.

In any given person some of these symptoms may be more pronounced than in others, or may even be totally absent. In most people with ME there is a variable pattern in which symptoms are strongly noted for a time only to fade and then reappear, sometimes over a period of days or weeks, sometimes over a period of months or years.

Just how these symptoms are distributed in a group of people with ME can be judged by an analysis carried out by Dr Patrick Donovan in the USA, of the major symptoms of a group of 40 patients aged between 17 and 50 diagnosed as having ME.

30 per cent had arrived at their doctor with a chief complaint of fatigue (the others had this as a secondary complaint).

28 per cent were so incapacitated by the fatigue that they were virtually bedridden and unable to function.

60 per cent could function in the home or at work but felt unnaturally fatigued with no additional energy available for anything but essential tasks.

63 per cent observed that their energy levels fluctuated from extreme unnatural fatigue to almost normal.

60 per cent had recurrent sore throats.

80 per cent had recurrently aching muscles. (Half of those with aching muscles had to stop whatever they were doing because of this discomfort, whereas the other half were only aware of the severe aching when they rested after effort.)

83 per cent had recurrent headaches.

45 per cent observed the combination of symptoms of fatigue, muscle aches and sore throats.

78 per cent were depressed or had unusual mood changes.

73 per cent had sleep problems.

65 per cent found concentrating difficult or impossible.

60 per cent had symptoms of anxiety.

55 per cent had symptoms of nausea.

44 per cent had swollen lymph glands.

40 per cent approximately had stomach ache, diarrhoea, cough, loss of appetite, vomiting and/or a variety of other associated symptoms.

60 per cent noted that the condition had created stress problems at home or at work, and roughly the same proportion had themselves wondered whether the symptoms 'might just all be in my head'.

In their past medical history 26 per cent of these patients had been infected by Epstein-Barr virus (the 'cause' of mononucleosis or glandular fever), while 38 per cent had previous herpes infections and fully 53 per cent had a history of food or drug allergies or of hay fever.

In another study of 44 patients with ME, conducted by Dr Andrew Lockie, the following patterns were discovered:

Average age was 25 (ranging from 8 to 60).

Average duration of symptoms when first seen by the doctor was 35 months (longest 15 years, shortest 6 weeks).

52 per cent had a history of glandular fever before the onset of symptoms.

81 per cent reported major emotional upsets in the six months before their condition began, mostly connected with break-up of relationships.

13 per cent believed the condition followed on from operations or accidents.

20 per cent believed it followed from vaccination.

Scientific Verification

Over the past few years research in earnest has begun on this condition in many medical centres, and to the relief of those previously labelled as neurotic or hysterical some concrete results have been produced. In *some* but not all people with ME clinical evidence has now shown the following:

- Raised serum levels of antibodies to Epstein-Barr virus, Coxsackie-B viruses or cytomegalovirus – in between 50 and 70 per cent of people with ME.
- A fall in T-helper lymphocytes (essential part of immune response).
- Disturbed muscle membrane conduction – in 75 per cent of those examined by electromyography.
- Abnormally increased acidification of muscles – seen in over 80 per cent of those tested, using magnetic resonance testing.
- A unique metabolic derangement in energy production in muscle cells shown by magnetic resonance investigation.
- Enterovirus particles in muscle tissues – found in about 25 per cent of people with ME.

Clearly there exists at present no absolute test for 'proving' the existence of a physical component of ME in *all* people thus affected. And even in those cases where such physical indicators are found, we should be cautious about concluding that these signs (antibodies, virus particles etc.) are necessarily causative, for they may themselves be symptoms of, or the result of, the underlying condition. In later chapters I will discuss this more fully, and will also examine some of the available tests and their implications.

Controversy often surrounds the discussion of ME. It is an emotive subject, witness headlines such as:

' "Yuppie Flu" Is All in the Mind, Say Doctors.' (*Sunday Times*, 10 July 1988)

'An Illness Doctors Don't Recognise.' (*Observer*, 1 June 1986)

'Gaining Credence: The Disease That Isn't Just in the Mind.' (*Daily Telegraph*, 28 July 1987)

'All in the Mind – or in the Body Too?' (*Daily Telegraph*, 19 July 1988)

After fifty years of investigation of ME by the medical profession there is still a continuing debate between those who insist that ME is nothing but a form of hysteria, a sort of exaggerated neurotic condition, and those who claim it to be rooted in causes of organic/physical/biochemical origin related directly to immune system depression.

In truth it may well be that both schools of thought are right, for the evidence derived from the very recent research work into the relationship between the mind and the immune system indicates a profound link between our beliefs, attitudes and mental/emotional habits, and the efficiency of the immune system. This area of study is called psychoneuroimmunology and it provides strong clues as to a link between depressed immune function, such as exists in true ME, and the mind of the person affected. This will be examined in detail in Chapter 3.

If it can be established that the effects of coping poorly with stress, anxiety and major 'life events', are potentially immune suppressing, then we might see that the 'hysteria' ('it's all in the mind') and the 'immune suppression' ('it's organic in origin') views are both valid. This could also provide us with a guide to the ways in which the problem should be treated, and prevented from recurring.

It is partly poor awareness of this powerful link between

the immune system and the mind which explains the confusion and emotion which this condition has generated both among the medical profession and the public.

No one wishes to have themselves labelled as 'neurotic' or hysterical. Bad enough that life for between 100,000 and 150,000 people in the UK alone is a struggle from morning to night. That getting out of bed and dressing is an effort as exhausting as climbing a mountain. That almost all mental and physical work is impossible because of a virtually total lack of energy reserves and a constant flu-like lethargy, malaise and muscular discomfort. To have added to such symptoms the allegation that this is a 'shirker's disease', merely evidence of a subconscious desire to opt out of normal life, is to compound the problem enormously.

These symptoms are, it has been pointed out by sceptics, merely the normal end-result of depression. Those afflicted will tell you, however, that the symptoms are so profoundly soul-destroying that depression is often a result, rather than the cause, of ME.

Again a combination of both viewpoints may be accurate in some cases. These are the words of M.L., a senior nursing officer and one of my patients, who was obliged to accept early retirement as a result of her ME: 'A year after the first symptoms I still feel very ill at times and exhausted. I often fall asleep during the day and when I wake up I cannot move or speak. I am still aware of surroundings and can understand what is being said. I sometimes have to use a wheelchair. This illness has totally turned our lives upside down.'

Another voice is that of Celia Wookey, a former general practitioner who was unable to continue medical practice because of her ME: 'For more than twenty years my own life has been dominated by this baffling and dispiriting illness, which drains both muscle and brain of energy. As with others my disease has waxed and waned, but eventually I had to give up both driving and my work as a GP. Despite my background I have been through the gamut of medical disbelief, including being diagnosed as suffering from hysteria.'

In these two cries from the heart we have encapsulated a number of the most common symptoms associated with ME. Exhaustion so profound that movement seems impossible is one. This distinctive sign of exhaustion on effort, as with most of the symptoms of the condition, waxes and wanes, comes and goes, is intermittent and variable in intensity for no apparent reason.

Both these quoted comments are from women who had medical backgrounds and this is also significant, for more women than men have ME and a surprising number have worked for many years in medically related professions. Not surprisingly, when these virtually disabling symptoms are met with disbelief, there is anguish and ultimately often profound depression which of course aggravates the condition.

Where Does the Truth Lie?

Based on the evidence to hand it seems clear that the causes of ME include elements of both stress-induced immune incompetence and a combination of possible associated symptom-producing factors, including all or any of the following:

- Hyperventilation and its associated biochemical changes and emotional symptoms.
- Recurrent or persistent bacterial or viral infection.
- Candida albicans overgrowth (a yeast parasite living in all of us).
- Nutritional deficiency.
- Toxic accumulations (often of heavy metals such as lead or mercury, or of pesticide residues).

11

- Hypoglycaemia.
- Environmental and food sensitivities and allergies.
- Inadequate energy synthesis.
- Hormonal imbalances.

By addressing all and any of these often-interacting components in any given case, as well as giving attention to the enormously important element of 'coping skills' (how you handle stress and the problems of life), a positive resolution of ME is almost always possible.

The good news then is that ME is curable, but largely by the endeavours of the person with ME, aided by a variety of methods and substances. The bad news is that it takes time, patience and often considerable personal effort.

In subsequent chapters I intend to examine those factors which have allowed ME to become so common in modern society. They comprise a complex and interwoven series of physical and mental/emotional factors which require attention if normal health is to be restored.

We are all unique genetically, biochemically, structurally, psychologically and emotionally, and we vary vastly and in many ways in our needs and potentials. It is a fundamental principle of healing that the individual who has a condition should be treated and not the condition which the individual 'has'. The interlocking causative elements operating in one person with ME may not be the same as those operating in someone else with ME.

This makes uniform prescriptions relating to nutrition, exercise, coping skills, etc. both unwise and indeed useless. We all require individual assessment of our needs and it may take a degree of trial and error in certain areas to find exactly what it is that suits you or what it is that meets your needs. In the chapters on the healing of ME, suggested options will be given for just this reason.

Another basic and inescapable truth is that the body is

self-healing and this is often taken for granted to such an extent that we overlook the importance of the fact. You know that you will heal if you cut yourself or even if in major trauma you break a bone. This self-healing process is constant, in good health.

However, if nutritional deficiencies exist; if toxic materials are absorbed from food or the atmosphere; if the ability to handle stress is poor or inadequate; if inborn idiosyncrasies create imbalances and demands which are not being met; if allergies or infections persist and if drugs have been used in treating these which cause further damage to internal ecology; if lifestyle habits are life-endangering rather than life-enhancing (smoking, inadequate sleep, poor home or work conditions, etc.); if all or any of these and numerous other possible factors are present, they require correction before the homoeostatic (self-healing) mechanisms on which all healing depends can operate and health can be restored.

It should be clear that the solution to health problems of this sort does not lie in 'magic bullets', in 'instant cures', and certainly not in methods or medications which ignore all the various causes and which attempt simply to obliterate the symptoms.

ME is 'curable' only by the concerted efforts of the person with ME, harnessing the self-healing potential of mind and body and simultaneously removing from the scene the elements which are preventing this from operating efficiently. This is not to say that support and help are not available, for they are, but it is important to realize that ultimately the body only heals itself when the opportunity to do so is present.

This, then, is our objective as together we seek those causes which may be operating in you, and look for ways in which support can be provided for your self-healing systems and mechanisms. Some of the healing methods will relate to the mind, the emotions and to stress-coping abilities. Others will relate to the physical enhancement of the body through nutrition and other approaches, which reduce susceptibility to infection and which enhance energy and immune function. We need to emphasize and involve both the mind and the body in order to restore health when ME is present.

REFERENCES

'All in the Mind – or in the Body Too?' Wookey, C., *Daily Telegraph*, 19 July 1988, p. 13.

'Chronic Enterovirus Infection in Patients with PVFS', Yousef, G., *et al.*, *The Lancet*, 23 January 1988, pp. 146–9.

'Postviral Fatigue Syndrome: Time for a New Approach', David, A., *et al.*, *British Medical Journal*, vol. 296, 5 March 1988, pp. 696–699.

Textbook of Natural Medicine, Pizzorno, J., Murray, M., JBCNM, Seattle 1987.

Tiredness and Fatigue, Shepherd, C., *GP*, May 1986, pp. 25–36.

'What Is ME?', Lloyd, A., *et al.*, *The Lancet*, 4 June 1988, pp. 1286–1287.

2 The Virus Connection: Cause or Consequence?

In many people with ME there is currently, or has been in the past, a demonstrably high level of virus activity. This is beyond question, as is the fact that such viral activity is not related to any particular virus, but rather to one of several which have been implicated, including Epstein-Barr virus, cytomegalovirus and a group known as Coxsackie-B viruses.

A major area of contention is whether such viral infection, in the past or present, is the result of, or the cause of, the various mental and emotional symptoms so often associated with ME.

The problem in trying to make such a judgment is that both viewpoints are probably accurate, with some of the susceptibility towards this type of viral infection being the result of an immune system compromised by a particular cluster of predisposing psychological attitudes and behavioural patterns. It is clear also of course that ME, once established, is the cause of a multitude of emotion- and mood-altering changes.

Pamela Holmes, writing in *Cosmopolitan*, says, 'It may be that the immune system of the ME sufferer has been "weakened" by circumstances or an individual's attitude and when this changes, recovery is possible.' She points out that, 'Young, ambitious women are more prone to ME, hence the term "yuppie flu" which is used in the States. In fact, people of all ages and sexes get ME. Dr Belinda Dawes [herself afflicted with ME], says there is an ME personality, "a fighter, who is determined to beat the disease. Unfortunately, that is precisely the attitude which has to change." Many people with ME have to learn to pace themselves even when they are feeling well.'

It will become clear as we examine the various factors which appear to be operating in people with ME that both its cause and cure involve no single element but rather a combination of interacting factors, ranging through nutritional deficits, candida albicans (yeast) overgrowth in the bowel, poor coping abilities in relation to stress and a possible consequent tendency to hyperventilation, as well as viral infection(s) sometimes made more likely because of 'attitude' or personality factors.

Dr Mark Hughson, writing in the *British Medical Journal*, points out that some doctors seem to fail to distinguish between emotional problems resulting from organic sources and emotional upset which is the result of being ill (with ME). He disagrees with the emphasis which claims that psychological changes may cause the disease. 'In patients known to me they result from it.'

This often confusing distinction between what causes and what is caused by the illness is a recurrent theme surfacing in most research related to ME. Further confusion is obvious when the virus connection is examined. In the US Epstein-Barr virus (EBV) has attracted the majority of the attention in relation to postviral fatigue. Indeed the condition is widely known as chronic Epstein-Barr syndrome. In the UK this common organism is also spoken of in relation to ME, but others such as cytomegalovirus and Coxsackie-B viruses are equally labelled as 'the cause'.

Epstein-Barr Virus

This is one of a group known as herpes viruses. These viruses seem to be able to take up residence in our bodies, secreting themselves and lying dormant until immune function is depressed thus allowing them to operate actively again for a while.

The cycle of dormant stage alternating with active stage is well known in people who are infected with herpes simplex (cold sore) virus, which reappears with its characteristic blisters or vesicles whenever the defences of the body are depressed (just before a new infection such as a cold for example, or after sunbathing – an immune suppressor – or at the time of menstruation). EBV follows a similar pattern of intermittent alternation between periods of quiescent and active behaviour, but without the blisters and vesicles.

By the time they reach adulthood most if not all people have been infected by EBV, which then takes refuge in the salivary glands and in the B-lymphocytes (part of the immune system's army of helping cells). If infection with EBV takes place in childhood no obvious symptoms may be seen. When, however, infection occurs in adolescence or early adult life approximately half of those infected have the characteristic symptoms of glandular fever (infectious mononucleosis).

The symptoms of infectious mononucleosis, which seems to be most common in people between the ages of fifteen and twenty-five, include headache, malaise (flu-like symptoms), fever, aching muscles, sore throat and swollen lymph glands (especially those on the side of the neck), a skin rash (sometimes) and of course extreme fatigue. A common additional symptom is an enlarged liver, and tests of liver function frequently show this organ to be operating poorly for some weeks after infection with EBV.

It is not hard to see why those doctors investigating ME have been drawn to call it a form of chronic EBV infection, since almost all the symptoms of the acute form are characteristic of postviral fatigue syndrome. Many American scientists strongly believe that ME is nothing more than chronic mononucleosis.

Is EBV Infectious?

In close contact, such as kissing, EBV is highly infectious in most people for up to six months after the initial acute infection, since saliva is one of the major fluids carrying this virus. Even when no symptoms of glandular fever are observed a small proportion of those infected (around a quarter) continue to be infectious, and this is especially true of people whose immune systems are compromised. Studies in the USA have demonstrated a persistently high level of EBV antibody activity in many patients with the symptoms of ME.

New Daily Persistent Headache Syndrome

A recent British study examined women suffering from persistent daily headaches which had developed suddenly and for no apparent reason. They found very high levels of antibody to EBV and state, 'The syndrome of headaches, fatigue and depression is commonly seen in clinical practice and is often attributed to neurosis. In some cases these symptoms are associated with serological evidence of EBV reactivation.'

The researchers question the role of the virus, saying that it is possible that the reactivation of EBV is 'secondary to stress and that stress precipitates transient immunosuppression'.

EBV virus was found in over 80 per cent of women with this 'new daily persistent headache' syndrome, which it seems from observation is very similar indeed to postviral fatigue syndrome (ME) since its associated symptoms are fatigue, depression, nausea, numb extremities and blurred vision (see Chapter 1 for list of ME symptoms).

Once again, as with cases diagnosed as ME, this virus is seen frequently to be part of the picture, but is it the cause or the result?

Cytomegalovirus

This is another micro-organism which can produce almost the same symptoms as those associated with infection by EBV, and which is often associated with a condition very like, or indistinguishable from, infectious mononucleosis.

Unlike EBV, though, the age group most usually affected by cytomegalovirus is slightly older, between twenty and thirty. It also varies slightly in the symptom pattern observed, there being only rarely any sign of sore throat or swollen lymph glands in the neck.

Coxsackie-B Viruses

These are among a type of virus called enteroviruses which are found most commonly in the gastro-intestinal tract and which are associated with a range of diseases including poliomyelitis, meningitis and many upper respiratory infections.

Enteroviruses include among their seventy-odd members not only polio viruses (three different types) but also six which are classified in a group called Coxsackie-B viruses. These have been linked to ME, and studies in Britain have shown that almost a quarter of those people with ME can be shown to have enterovirus nucleic acid

(RNA) present in their muscles. Some of these people had been infected over twenty years previously, which strongly indicates the validity of the idea that such viral infections can remain either dormant or active in the body for a long long time.

A subsequent study at St Mary's Hospital Medical School, London, has confirmed that both faecal and serum samples of many people with a diagnosis of ME showed strong positive evidence of enterovirus infection, and that in the same people this evidence was again to be found a year later. Thus chronic infection with enteroviruses is clearly a part of the process in at least some ME patients.

An outbreak of ME occurred in the West of Scotland in 1980–1. Coxsackie-B virus antibody levels were found to be high in 60 per cent of those examined (22 patients), as opposed to only about 5 per cent of the general population.

Is this virus a cause, or part of a larger immune-compromised situation? The researchers investigating the Scottish outbreak observed that since sleep pattern disturbances, panic attacks, emotional sensitivity and poor concentration are all a part of the symptom picture of ME in many people, it would be of interest to investigate levels of Coxsackie-B virus in people undergoing psychiatric assessment for a variety of mental/emotional/psychological problems.

They therefore studied 247 such patients, both male and female. Of these 12.5 per cent had high Coxsackie-B virus antibody levels (compared with between 4 and 5 per cent in 'well' people). Interestingly they found that the percentage showing positive levels of this virus was highest in the psychiatric patients aged between thirty and thirty-nine.

In subsequent studies using very recent developments in research this same team showed that almost 40 per cent of patients diagnosed as having ME were displaying a reaction to Coxsackie-B viruses.

One significant characteristic of Coxsackie-B viruses is

their well known tendency to affect muscle tissue, a major problem area for ME sufferers. The researchers conclude: 'Although other virus infections, e.g. influenza, varicella, rubella, Epstein-Barr may precipitate ME, the data we have accumulated over the past six years suggest that Coxsackie-B viruses play an important role in the illness.'

Other Viruses

A suggestion is made by American researchers such as Dr Patrick Donovan that chronic infection by weakened live rubella virus given during vaccination could be responsible for chronic mononucleosis-like symptoms. This can apparently be passed to adults. There is a direct correlation between the degree of rubella antibody activity and mononucleosis-like symptoms. Rubella is not a serious disease and vaccination against it is largely performed in the hope of preventing the appearance of the disease during pregnancy where it can result in serious birth defects.

Over the years reports have been appearing in the medical press, mainly in the US, of vast numbers of children receiving this form of immunization who have suffered serious side-effects. *Science* (26 March 1977) states, 'The department of Health Education and Welfare reported that as many as 26 per cent of children receiving rubella vaccination in national programs developed arthralgia or arthritis.' In the *New England Journal of Medicine* (31 October 1985) a report appeared which was entitled 'Persistent Rubella Virus Infection Associated with Chronic Arthritis in Children'.

The connection between arthritis and ME is not clear. However it is known that, in any given form of infection, a wide range of degree exists in terms of both the symptoms and the intensity of those symptoms. Some people infected

21

by any virus or bacterium will suffer mild symptoms and others major ones. If arthritis appears in many children after rubella vaccination, may not milder symptoms (ME) appear in others? And if this is capable of transmission, is it not possible that adults in contact with such children could become affected?

Such virus activity has been established as long as eight years after initial vaccination, although the person had had a normal immune response to the vaccination. This suggests that the immune response was insufficient to obliterate the viral activity, which simply continued over the years, producing the arthritic symptoms, or possibly milder muscular dysfunction and fatigue. It is often possible to isolate such viruses from the joints of children and adults affected by arthritis, implicating them in some of the inflammatory reactions in such joints.

The ME connection is at least worthy of investigation.

Immune System Involvement

The implication of continuing viral activity of any sort is that it will ultimately disturb the efficiency of the immune system. In one study of 50 unexplained cases of acute or chronic fatigue fully 35 were found to have altered immune function relating to their lymphocytes, key elements of the defence system. It was considered by the researchers that these abnormalities related to persisting Epstein-Barr virus activity. Other studies have shown variations in immune dysfunction.

Again we come across the same vexed question of whether these people were not also in some way compromising their immune systems through their psychological patterns, and the studies I have mentioned above have been strongly criticized because they ignored this psychological dimension. It seems that we cannot doubt the fact that immune function will be depressed if viral activity continues. However, we cannot know whether the viral activity is not actually allowed to persist because of immune suppression resulting from, or influenced by, emotional or psychological causes. Or do any psychological changes such as depression merely result from the effects of viral activity and the multitude of unpleasant symptoms which follow?

As we will discover in Chapter 3 psychological stress clearly can produce immune suppression, as can sleep deprivation and an imbalanced diet. In one study using animals it was found that infection with Coxsackie-B virus only occurred when environmental stress was operating. Is it not most likely that sometimes a mixture of both elements, psychological stress and viral activity, is present and that the best therapeutic approach should take account of this?

In people with AIDS and AIDS-related complex (ARC) the symptom pattern is very similar to that seen in severe ME, although obviously there is a great difference in degree. Doctors at Harvard Medical School have recently questioned seriously whether ARC is not a severe form of what they call chronic Epstein-Barr virus syndrome, since EBV is found to be (or to have been) active in almost all such patients.

Patrick Donovan asks, 'The relationship between abnormal EBV serological (blood fluids) tests in immuno-compromised states or immunologically related diseases raises many questions about the involvement of EBV and these diseases. Is EBV a causative agent creating an immunologically compromised or disrupted state, or is its reactivation a manifestation of a previously existing mal-functioning immune system?'

He acknowledges that this important, almost funda-mental question, is hard to answer but that a recent report in the *Journal of the American Medical Association* concludes, 'some patients with these illnesses (syndromes of chronic fatigue) may have an abnormality of infectious and/or immunological origin'.

In one study (involving 134 patients) not only were EBV antibody levels found to be high but also levels of antibodies to cytomegalovirus and herpes simplex viruses types 1 and 2, as well as to measles virus. This could only be happening in someone with a compromised immune system, and the combination of infections (almost certainly accompanied by yeast overgrowth – see 'The Candida-ME Link', Chapter 6) would be constantly devitalizing and sapping what immune function remained intact.

Is it any wonder that fatigue and a host of other symptoms would be manifest in a person so compromised, or that the individual might well become depressed?

Looking again at the AIDS model we can see resemblances in the way in which multiple contributory elements have allowed the condition to develop. One of the leading researchers into viral activity, Professor Peter Duesberg of the University of California, Berkeley, stated in the *New Scientist*, 28 April 1988 (in relation to the way AIDS develops), 'Multiple factors, such as viral and microbial infections or non-infectious toxins, may therefore cause these symptoms.'

If we look at the way ME develops, the same statement applies, only to this list we could add nutritional deficiencies as well as psychological stress (and indeed these should be on the list of factors contributing to AIDS onset as well).

The Revici Hypothesis

Emanuel Revici is a medical doctor practising in New York. He is in his early nineties and has been a powerful force in trying to establish biological methods of treating both cancer and AIDS. In doing so he has, over the years, researched the ways in which natural checks and balances on bacterial, fungal and viral micro-organisms work in nature.

Dr Revici has noted that in the process of evolution, from very simple organisms to more complex ones, a biological 'hierarchy' has evolved. Each slightly more evolved, more complex, organism has assured itself of at least some degree of protection from the less developed organisms which preceded it in evolutionary terms.

In this hierarchy we have at the very bottom of the scale viruses, followed by bacteria and then fungi, going on eventually to plant life and animals. We are all aware that fungal extracts kill bacteria, and it is well established that a variety of plant extracts are antifungal.

Revici reasoned therefore that bacterial micro-organisms would have a powerful antiviral potential. He says, 'In the progressive development of the biological realm, a more complex formation has its life and autonomy assured only if it can resist the noxious action exerted by the inferior entities in the series. I thus recognized that a natural defence exists between levels. For example, microbes defend against viruses, and fungi defend against microbes (as witness the existence of a wide range of antimicrobial antibiotics derived from fungi).'

He then studied the ways in which microbes defend themselves against virus activity and found that the major antiviral activity was found in their use of fatty acids and proteins from their nuclei. This research continues, but knowledge of it encourages the use of 'natural' bacterial cultures such as lactobacillus acidophilus – a type of naturally occurring 'friendly' bacteria which lives in all of us unless destroyed by antibiotics – as a means of re-establishing control over viruses which live in our digestive tracts, including the enteroviruses such as Coxsackie-B. Other antiviral methods derive from Revici's work, as we shall see in Chapter 11 which looks at the ways in which we can assist the defences of the body in this direction. These biological methods are safe and have no side-effects.

Medical Treatment of Virus Infections

Most medical treatment of virus infection involves powerful drugs which, while having antiviral potential, also usually have a variety of associated side-effects, one of which is often a further depression of immune function. AZT, currently the only drug used in treating persistent viral activity in AIDS patients, is just such a one.

One recent medical discovery is the function of a substance called interferon. Its use by doctors to treat viral infections has resulted in a fascinating possibility, that interferon is the cause of at least some of the symptoms of ME.

The Interferon Hypothesis: Is This the Cause of the Symptoms of ME?

Interferons are proteins made by our cells as the first line of defence in response to viral attack. They serve to inhibit the multiplication of many viruses.

When interferon (IFN) was first synthesized and used as a medication to try to boost the defence of the body against viral infection, such as the common cold, it seemed to work quite well for many people but produced unpleasant side-effects such as fatigue, headache, malaise etc. which often made the treatment worse than the condition being treated.

In order to see whether the symptoms of ME might not be resulting from too much IFN a study was undertaken by doctors in London (by a gentle irony, from the Royal Free Hospital) and Wales.

They reasoned that since the symptoms of ME resemble those seen when interferon (IFN) is used therapeutically this hypothesis was quite likely to be correct. They noted that when the same idea had been considered previously, elevated levels of IFN had been sought in the bloodstreams of people with chronic ME, but without success. Once again the spectre of 'what is real ME?' was raised, for the doctors involved in this study maintain that, 'there is a lack of an objective clinical marker to distinguish genuine cases from patients with other complaints such as minor neuro-psychiatric disease'.

This problem, they say, is less obvious when children with ME are examined, and so they investigated the levels of IFN produced by children from a school in Wales where there had been a recent outbreak of ME. In all they investigated eight affected children and the parents of one of the children. Of the children, four had persistent symptoms of over three months' duration and the other four had recovered after at least five months of the illness. All those still affected had profound fatiguability and malaise, as well as a variety of symptoms ranging from chest pains to sore throats and visual problems. Other children in the same classes, who had not been affected by ME, were also assessed for their levels of IFN production. *The findings showed that in response to a viral stimulus the cells of these children (both still ill and recovered) produced significantly excessive levels of Alpha-IFN as compared with children who had not had ME.*

Does this mean that we now know the cause of the symptoms of ME? Possibly for some of them, in some people, but it does not answer the question, why do these people produce too much IFN? Is it not possible that the over-production of IFN is the result of a generally depleted immune function in which over-compensation occurs as the remnants of immune defence try to slow the infection?

27

If persistent or recurrent viral activity exists, this is due to a failure of the normal defences to deal with the problem, for any of the reasons we are looking at in this section (nutritional, stress-induced etc.). In such a situation excessive IFN production can be seen to be quite natural. The answer would seem to lie in enhancement of the other elements of immune function, along with efforts to retard or eliminate the viral interloper without further weakening the system – as do most current medical antiviral strategies. IFN over-production is itself a symptom – not a cause.

Are There Safer Alternatives to Medical Treatment?

Yes there are, and these include three strategies. One is nutritional and will be discussed in Chapter 9, where we will examine possible nutritional approaches to enhancing immune function.

A second involves specific herbal products which have known antiviral properties without side-effects. This will be explained in Chapter 11 which deals with anti-candida and antiviral methods.

In that chapter we will also look at another strategy in which substances can be used which increase the resistance to infection of the cells of the body. One of these is called AL721, and it is basically a mixture of different lipids (oils and fats) derived largely from egg yolks, and constituted in a specific ratio (7:2:1). The AL stands for active lecithin and this was researched initially at the Weizmann Institute in Israel and discussed in major texts dealing with what is known as 'membrane engineering', in which the membranes of the cells of the body (their outer covering) are strengthened, thus reducing the chance of infection. This method is in accord with Revici's hypothesis.

There is a viral connection with ME in most cases, although we may never be sure whether this is the cause or a consequence of the process. Such ignorance, however, should not stop us from trying to eliminate the continuing viral drain on limited immune resources, while at the same time dealing with anything else which may be further reducing immune competence, such as stress and nutritional imbalances.

REFERENCES

'AIDS and the "Innocent" Virus', Duesberg, P., *New Scientist*, 28 April 1988, pp. 34–5.

'Chronic Enterovirus Infection in Patients with Postviral Fatigue Syndrome', Yousef, G., *et al.*, *The Lancet*, 23 January 1988, pp. 146–9.

'Chronic Mononucleosis-Like Syndrome', Donovan, P., chapter in *Textbook of Natural Medicine* by Pizzorno, J. and Murray, M., JBCNM, Seattle 1987.

'Coxsackie-B Viruses and Myalgic Encephalomyelitis', Bell, E., *et al.*, *Journal of Royal Society of Medicine*, vol. 81, no. 6, June 1988, pp. 329–31.

Immunization Related Syndrome, Snead, E., monograph, Metro Medical Publications, San Antonio, Texas 1987.

'Increased Frequency of EBV Excretion in Patients with New Daily Persistent Headaches', Diaz-Mitoma, F., *et al.*, *The Lancet*, 21 February 1987, pp. 411–14.

'Interferon Production in Postviral Fatigue Syndrome', Lever, A., *et al.*, correspondence, *The Lancet*, 9 July 1988, p. 101.

'Is AIDS a Form of Epstein-Barr Virus Disease?' Otleb, C., report in *New York Native*, 27 July 1987.

'M.E. and You', Holmes, P., *Cosmopolitan*, February 1988, pp. 91–94.

'Persistent Rubella Virus Infection Associated with Chronic Arthritis in Children', *New England Journal of Medicine*, vol. 313, no. 18, 31 October 1985, p. 1117.

'Postviral Fatigue Syndrome', Hughson, M., correspondence,

British Medical Journal, vol. 296, 9 April 1988, p. 1067.

'Postviral Fatigue Syndrome: Persistence of Enterovirus RNA in Muscle and Elevated Creatine Kinase', Archard, L., *et al.*, *Journal of Royal Society of Medicine*, vol. 81, no. 6, June 1988, pp. 326–8.

'Postviral Fatigue Syndrome: Time for a New Approach', David, A., *et al.*, *British Medical Journal*, vol. 296, 5 March 1988, pp. 696–699.

'Research and Theoretical Background for Treatment of AIDS', Revici, E., *Townsend Letter for Doctors*, Feb./March 1987, issue 45, pp. 1–13.

Vaccination, Immunisation: Dangers, Delusions and Alternatives, Chaitow, L., C. W. Daniel, Saffron Walden 1987.

3 The Mind, the Immune System and ME

Dr David Smith is a medical doctor employed by the ME society in the United Kingdom. In an address to this association in 1985 he said: 'One observation of mine is that nearly 100 per cent of those who develop the postviral fatigue syndrome were, before their virus infection, under a great deal of stress and I think that this question of stress load certainly suggests – from my point of view – that there was a predisposing factor in the people who were under an enormous amount of psychological, work or marriage stress, or whatever type of stress it was. They seem to be more influenced to get this disease process than those who were not [stressed].'

Dr Andrew Lockie is a medical doctor who uses mainly homoeopathic medicine. At a workshop on fatigue in London in 1988 he presented a breakdown of the pre-disposing causes of forty of his patients with ME. No fewer than 81 per cent had had major emotional/psychological shocks in the months prior to the development of their illness. Most of these related to the breakup of relationships.

One of the major side-issues relating to ME is the

apparent susceptibility of members of the medical and associated professions. A large number of doctors and nurses have been affected and some of the main epidemics have taken place in hospitals. These include hundreds affected in Los Angeles (1934), the outbreak at Harefield Sanatorium in England (1939), 140 affected in Durban (1955), and of course one of the most discussed outbreaks, in which 292 members of staff and 12 patients at the Royal Free Hospital in London were affected, also in 1955.

Doctors and nurses are subject to a great deal of stress and often to impossibly difficult working hours (twenty-four hours non-stop is far from unusual), and a well researched phenomenon which affects such people – as well as high-powered executive types – is known as 'burn-out'. This self-explanatory term leads to virtual inability to function, often to increased use of stimulants such as alcohol, and unfortunately all too often to suicide. Such people would certainly fit well into Dr Smith's 'people under a great deal of stress prior to developing ME'.

The Royal Free episode led to an investigation, using the case cards of those affected. The report on this research by Drs McEvedy and Beard appeared in 1970 and has been the source of debate and anger ever since.

People with ME who have sought and claimed a physical cause for ME (virus for example) reject out of hand the suggestion by McEvedy and Beard that the Royal Free episode (and by implication all other cases of ME) was an example of 'epidemic hysteria'. They see the associated emotional and psychological phenomena as being the result, rather than a cause of, ME.

This defensive attitude was summed up by Dr David Poskanzer of the Harvard Medical School when he replied to the report by McEvedy and Beard: 'Instead of ascribing . . . ME to mass hysteria or psychoneurosis, may I suggest that the authors consider the possibility that all psychoneurosis is a residual deficit from epidemic or sporadic cases of ME.'

Perhaps the term 'mass hysteria' is an unfortunate one and this may have resulted in the baby being thrown out with the bathwater, since it has led to a widespread tendency to reject any suggestion of a psychological or personality factor in the sequence of events which leads to ME. This is doubly unfortunate because it is only through the recognition that there is often – though by no means always – just such a component, as well as a variety of associated 'physical' causes acting in concert, that a real understanding of ME can be achieved, and via this a rational and successful treatment programme developed.

It would seem to any reasonable observer that the overall classification of ME should contain subgroups which indicate which factors seem to predominate in the condition of a particular individual. Such subgroups might include those with obvious psycho-social elements; those which clearly follow on from a viral infection or which can be shown to involve persistent or recurrent viral activity; and those which have as a major element an allergic component.

Of course in any of such subgroups the likelihood is that there will be a large degree of overlap, especially since each of these three subgroups (psychological, allergy and viral infection) can be shown to be capable of strongly influencing both of the others.

The Mind–Immune System Connection

In a leading article in *The Lancet* (27 June 1987) this connection was examined in the light of the most recent research. Among the fascinating evidence which has emerged are the results of studies involving healthy young volunteers as well as students at exam time and patients suffering a variety of psychiatric conditions.

All point clearly and definitively to an inescapable fact, that the immune system is capable of being massively depressed in one or other of its multiple roles, by psychological factors.

The Lancet discussion tells us that one aspect of a normal immune system's response to an invading micro-organism (an antigen) is for blood lymphocytes to undergo an alteration to what is called a blastogenic form. This is termed simply the mitogen response. This response has been widely reported to decrease when the person is depressed, and to return to normal when the depression goes.

Similar changes in immune response have been observed in people affected by major changes in their lives (known as 'life events' to doctors). Other changes seen when depression is current include a decrease in the absolute number of elements of the immune system such as lymphocytes, B-cells and T-cells.

A common way of testing immune function is to assess the activity of what are called natural killer cells, which kill tumour cells rapidly and which are an important part of the body's first line of defence. Natural killer cell activity (NKCA) was measured in undergraduates who were reporting psychological distress in relation to previous life events. Their NKCA was compared with that of other undergraduates who had had similar life event shocks but who reported no psychological distress. It was found that in the 'poor copers' the NKCA was lower than that found in the 'good copers'.

This suggested that stress in itself was not a cause of immune suppression, but that the coping ability (therefore the psychology and personality) of the person decided whether shocks and strain in life would have this depressing immune effect.

In other studies medical students were examined for

emotional stress reactions to loneliness and at examination time, as well as having their NKCA monitored. The findings showed that psychological well-being was associated with good NKCA, while poor NKCA was evident in less psychologically healthy individuals.

The Lancet editorial concludes, after examining this and other evidence, 'This implies that it is the individual's response to stress that determines the effect on immunity, rather than the stress itself.'

Another undesirable response to stress can be a tendency to hyperventilate. The tendency to overbreathe (and to over-exhale) dramatically alters the chemistry of the blood as excessive quantities of carbon-dioxide are breathed out. In turn, this has profound psychological and neurological effects, as will become clear in Chapter 4 which deals with the subject. Most of the symptoms seen in hyperventilation are also common to people suffering from ME.

This further strengthens a putative link between the mind and at least some cases of ME, since it can now be shown that poor coping ability can result not only in depressed immune function – leading inevitably to an increased likelihood of infection (or of reactivated viral activity) – but also in the production of many of the symptoms so demoralizing to the ME patient.

A further ramification of this complex of changes relating to stress is that when the immune system is upset by stress reactions, allergies become more likely (allergy is simply an over-response of the immune system to a foreign substance). Many cases of ME have been shown to be helped by dealing with an allergic tendency. This will be explained in Chapter 5.

The evidence presented above, of the connection between aspects of the depression of the immune system and emotional distress, falls short of actual proof that this necessarily results in viral infection. Such evidence is, however, to hand and specifically relates to ME since it deals with infection by Epstein-Barr virus leading to glandular fever (mononucleosis) which is discussed fully in Chapter 2.

Researchers at the University of Colorado presented evidence in *Psychology Today* of a clear link between the mind and this specific viral infection.

Samples of blood were taken from all cadets entering West Point Military Academy to discover which of them had previously been exposed to Epstein-Barr virus infection. Of those students not previously infected, and therefore vulnerable to such infection since they had no antibodies to the virus, about a fifth developed mononucleosis each year. The other susceptible students were assumed to have more efficient immune systems which prevented full-blown EBV infection from developing.

Psychological profiles were performed on all the susceptible students and it was found that most of those who did develop mononucleosis had one particular trait which was summarized as desperately wishing for a military career but being basically underachievers and therefore developing anxiety in response to the perceived stress. These students actually made their immune systems more vulnerable because of their anxiety and 'allowed' EBV to infect them as a result.

What Are Good Coping Skills?

It has been observed that in certain professions stress-related illness is extremely high. Air traffic controllers are one such group and study of these overworked individuals has resulted in some fascinating evidence, for not all air traffic controllers are made ill by the stress and unnatural working hours involved in their job. Examination of how these 'good copers' manage to avoid stress-related illness shows that there exist a cluster of attitudes which together form what is known as the 'hardiness factor'.

This involves such elements as a feeling of control over one's environment (rather than feeling at the mercy of the fates), commitment to being involved in it (rather than feeling isolated and disconnected from events and people) and seeing the future as a challenge which will be successfully met rather than having a sense of apprehension towards it. I will expand on these themes in Chapter 10 which deals with harnessing mind-power in the healing process.

Psychoneuroimmunology

This new science deals with the effects of personality, stress and emotions on immune-associated diseases whether these involve infection, cancer, allergies or what are called autoimmune diseases where the body attacks itself (rheumatoid arthritis, colitis etc.).

The study of these connections developed from a somewhat surprising accidental observation. We are probably all familiar with Pavlov's dogs. These were the animals which this famous Russian scientist used in his experiments some sixty years ago to prove the existence of what he termed the 'conditioned reflex'. Having conditioned his dogs by ringing a bell before their food arrived, he then rang the bell without delivering the food. Not unnaturally the dogs had salivated before the arrival of their food and had associated the bell with this event. When the bell rang they continued to salivate even when no food appeared.

In a 1975 study of the sweetening agent Aspartame a doctor Robert Ader injected a group of rats with a drug meant to make them feel sick after they had consumed water in which Aspartame was dissolved thus, he hoped, making them dislike the sweet water.

They did indeed associate the effects of the injections with drinking the water, for even after these were stopped they dutifully became sick. Unfortunately, however, after a short while his rats began to die. Ader investigated and found that the drug he had been using in the initial injections was immunosuppressive.

Not only had the rats learned to be sick when they drank the water after the injections had ceased, they had learned to mimic identically the effects of that drug and continued to suppress their own immune functions to the point of dying. This was the first clear evidence of a controlling link between the mind and the immune system.

The study of what is now called psychoneuroim-munology, which has developed from this original accidental observation, clearly shows a two-way link between the immune system and the brain, involving both the nervous system and hormonal secretions. Disturbances in one of these areas affects the others, and emotional upsets and distress alter the incidence, severity and course of ill-health and disease (though much of this is modified by personality factors and coping skills).

Severe emotional disturbance is almost always associated with a depressed immune function. The comedian Woody Allen has summed this up in a sentence, 'I don't get depressed; I grow a tumour instead.'

A Medical Problem

A problem exists in medicine in which if a condition has a 'psychological' label it tends to attract little interest from general physicians. An article previously referred to, from the *British Medical Journal* of 5 March 1988 (entitled 'Postviral Fatigue Syndrome: Time for a New Approach'), highlights this: 'Most accounts of the postviral fatigue syndrome acknowledge the universal presence of psychological disturbances, ranging from mild depression or anxiety to severe behavioural abnormalities. . . . There has been little systematic investigation of psychiatric features and no distinctive pattern of symptoms has emerged . . . Though collaboration among virologists, histopathologists, neurologists and general practitioners is to be commended, the failure of more psychiatrists (other than those interested in mass hysteria) to contribute leaves a yawning gap in this research.'

This article goes on to ask the question, 'Why have sufferers and their doctors been so vigorous in rejecting the possibility that these ubiquitous psychological factors may be aetiological (causative) in their postviral fatigue syndrome?'

The authors conclude that this is because patients have encountered unhelpful and even hostile responses from doctors who hold that psychological illness is not 'real' illness. Their humiliation is linked in the minds of many such patients with the 'psychological' label. This reflects, says the article, very badly on both doctors and on psychiatrists, who have failed to get the message of their science across to the public and their fellow-members of the medical profession.

It is, in the authors' view, only by means of a non-judgmental approach which recognizes the mind/body link that progress will be made. The irony of course is that so many members of that profession are themselves ME sufferers.

A corollary to the idea that immune function can be depressed by negative psychological and emotional states is that the opposite is also true. This can be stated clearly as, 'Enhancement of immunity can also be conditioned.' In other words we can learn to make our immune systems more efficient by learning positive, life-enhancing strategies which improve the hardiness factor and our ability to cope with the vicissitudes of life.

A variety of behavioural strategies including psycho-therapy, relaxation techniques, meditation, guided imagery (visualization), biofeedback, hypnosis etc. can all be shown to optimize immune function. George Solomon, one of the pioneer scientists involved in psychoneuroimmunology, says, 'If noxious effects (such emotions as anxiety, grief, depression and loneliness) are immunosuppressive, then it stands to reason that whatever psychotherapeutic or psychopharmacological intervention makes for a distress-free state of mind might be expected to improve immune function.'

The title of an article in the *Journal of the Royal College of Medicine* (June 1987) asks 'Are Happy People Healthier?' Solomon asks, 'Are happiness, security, sense of control, relaxation, and other positive emotions accompanied by immune enhancement?' The answer must be yes to both of these questions, and this is of profound importance to people with ME, as well as for all illnesses in which the immune function plays a major part.

None of the discussion in this chapter should create a defensive reaction in people with ME who are convinced of the 'physical' nature of their condition. It should, rather, help all of us to realize that the mind/body link is perhaps even stronger than we had ever imagined and that the evidence to hand indicates that this offers a powerful aid to recovery.

Of course, viral activity may require other methods of control as well. Of course other associated contributory elements such as allergy, nutritional deficiency, candida albicans overgrowth, negative life-style habits etc. may all need specific attention, but to neglect the power of the mind in relation to these things is to forego a major ally in the recovery effort.

It goes without saying, I hope, that the use of medication can only play a peripheral part in treating a condition with such multi-factorial causes and symptoms. To alter or mask the symptoms by the use of drugs is certainly no more than short-term palliation. Cure must come from within, and this requires immune enhancement, and removal of causes, by safe natural means.

REFERENCES

'Are Happy People Healthier?' Wood, C., *Journal of the Royal Society of Medicine*, vol. 80, June 1987, pp. 354–6.

'Depression, Stress and Immunity', editorial, *The Lancet*, 27 June 1987, pp. 1467–8.

'Emerging Field of Psychoneuroimmunology', Solomon, G., *Advances*, Institute for the Advancement of Health, vol. 2, no. 1, 1985, pp. 6–19.

'Lassitude', editorial, *British Medical Journal*, 20 April 1985, pp. 1161–2.

'Medical Addresses Given at 1985 ME Association AGM', reported in *Meeting Place #24*, the journal of the Australian and New Zealand ME Society, May 1986 edition.

'Postviral Fatigue Syndrome: Time for a New Approach', David, A., *et al.*, *British Medical Journal*, 5 March 1988, pp. 696–9.

'Stress and Health: Exploring the Links', Maier, S., Landenslager, M., *Psychology Today*, vol. 19, August 1985, pp. 44–9.

' "Yuppie Flu" Is All in the Mind, Say Doctors', Hodgkinson, N., *Sunday Times*, 17 July 1988, pp. 1–3.

4 Hyperventilation and ME

Many studies have concentrated on the widespread problem of over-breathing. Much of this research has related to its connection with anxiety states, in which it can lead to acute phobia accompanied by panic attacks of an incapacitating nature.

The effect of over-breathing is to reduce swiftly the levels of carbon-dioxide in the blood, altering the acid-alkaline balance and thus producing changes in the way nerves interact with each other. This results in a variety of unpleasant symptoms.

The symptoms most often associated with hyperventilation include giddiness, dizziness, faintness, numbness of the upper limbs, face or trunk, loss of consciousness, visual disturbance in which blurring or even temporary loss of vision is experienced, headaches of a general nature often accompanied by nausea and frequently diagnosed as migraine, inability to walk properly (ataxia) as well as trembling and head noises.

A number of symptoms often associated with heart function can become apparent during or after hyperventilation, including palpitation, chest discomfort, difficulty in taking a deep breath, insomnia, fatigue, weakness in the limbs and much more.

Of patients diagnosed with hyperventilation more than half are found to be undergoing stress, related to marriage, work or finance.

It should be clear that many of the problems experienced by the person who is hyperventilating are common to ME patients.

Hyperventilation is not, however, always associated with psychiatric stress and this is made clear in correspondence in the *Journal of the Royal Society of Medicine* (November 1987) in which it was stated that, 'The underlying disorder [of hyperventilation] may be psychiatric, organic, a habit disorder, or a combination of these.'

Approaches to Hyperventilation

In most instances of hyperventilation, a learned pattern of breathing comes into operation in response to real or assumed stressful situations. This over-breathing is usually found to co-exist alongside severely contracted muscles relating to the rib cage, the spinal regions and the diaphragm area.

We all tend to 'lock' our emotional states into our muscles. You only have to sit quietly and imagine a strong emotion such as fear or hatred or anger, for subtle yet perceptible changes to be felt in the muscles of the neck, shoulders, chest, pit of the stomach etc. If this were not just an imagined emotion but a strongly held one which lasted for many months or years, as is all too often the case, chronic shortening and tension would develop in many muscles of the body.

This state of affairs has two major implications for people with ME. One is that if muscles are chronically hypertonic, shortened or contracted, they cannot function normally, and this can usually be seen to be the case in people who hyperventilate. They have, it seems, 'learned' to over-breathe excessively in response to what are not really stressful situations.

In fact it is perfectly normal to hyperventilate when excessive demands are required of the body. Faced with a crisis our defence system prepares us for action instantly, and one of the mechanisms involved in this is an increase in available oxygen and an increase in clearance of carbon-dioxide through deeper, more rapid breathing. Were there to be a real crisis in which physical action such as running or fighting were involved, this reaction would be entirely appropriate and the hyperventilation would be part of a potentially life-saving response.

If, however, this response occurs inappropriately, in the face of a perceived but unreal crisis, such as exists when we are unnaturally anxious about something (this is a definition of a phobia), then the sequence of over-breathing would lead to imbalanced blood-gas levels, changes in acidity/alkalinity and the whole sequence of hyperventilation symptoms already listed.

Hyperventilation can become an habitual method of responding to all minor stress situations, leading to the complete misery of phobic states compounded by panic attacks and virtual incapacity and inability to function. Sufferers respond well to breathing re-training, and then learning to recognize that if they use their newly acquired slow breathing techniques in the face of a stressful (real or imagined) situation they can stop the symptoms because they will not hyperventilate. Some of the simple methods which can help towards this ideal will be outlined in Chapter 10.

A second result when muscles are held in a state of tension (due to emotional or other causes) for long periods is that enormous amounts of energy are wasted. The musculo-skeletal system is the largest energy-user in the body, and if major parts of it are working when they should be resting it is as wasteful of available energy as having many of the lights and power points in a house switched on when they are not required.

This may be an acceptable drain on energy if all is well and health is good. It is not an acceptable demand on the limited resources of someone whose energy reserves are depleted, as they are in ME.

One suggested method of reducing this drain is for people in a state of muscular tension to have regular access to bodywork. This could be in the form of massage (deep not surface stroking) or soft-tissue manipulation or osteopathic or chiropractic treatment.

The advantage of such care is that it both releases these long-held tensions and at the same time helps the regions thus affected to be able to function more normally. One such region is the rib cage, which if held in a state of rigidity cannot function normally even if the very best exercises are learned.

Correction of hyperventilation therefore should involve a threefold approach.

1 Learn *not* to respond to stress in the habitual way. This requires insights which may only be available from a good counsellor or psychotherapist. Relaxation techniques are a part of this.
2 Learn correct breathing techniques, for use especially when confronted by a frightening situation.
3 Normalize the machinery which governs breathing by bodywork and exercises. This conserves energy and allows normal function.

The result of such an approach is a lessened waste of energy, increased functional ability in relation to breathing, and far fewer symptoms.

Clearly, this is not the answer for everybody, and if it is the case that in most sufferers a variety of factors are present, with differing degrees of significance, then different therapeutic emphases are going to be required accordingly. Re-learning breathing methods would probably have only a small effect on candida; treatment of candida overgrowth would not be expected to do much for nutritional deficiencies; and so on. However, as part of an overall healing programme, the problem of hyperventilation should never be ignored.

REFERENCES

'Acute Chest Pain without Obvious Cause before Age 40 – Personality and Recent Life Events', Roll, M., *et al.*, *Journal of Psychosomatic Research*, vol. 31, no. 2, pp. 215–21.

'Anxiety and Muscle Tension Pain', Barlow, W., *British Journal of Clinical Practice*, May 1959, pp. 339–49.

'Enhanced Adaptive Behavioural Response in Agoraphobic Patients Pretreated with Breathing Retraining', Bonn, J., Readhead, C., *The Lancet*, 22 September 1984, pp. 665–8.

'Hyperventilation and Anxiety State', editorial, *Journal of Royal Society of Medicine*, vol. 74, January 1981, pp. 1–4.

'Respiratory and Psychiatric Abnormalities in Chronic Symptomatic Hyperventilation, Bass, C., Gardner, W., *British Medical Journal*, 11 May 1985, pp. 1387–90.

5 Allergy, Toxicity and ME

Many people with ME suffer from a wide range of environmental and food allergies and sensitivities. Such things as house dust, petrol fumes, perfumes and household cleaning substances can all produce violent reactions if the immune system is overresponding and the person has become sensitized to the chemicals in the substance. This is frequently the case in ME (especially if candida is active).

The obvious first strategy in such a situation is to avoid contact with or exposure to whatever it is that seems to be producing the reaction. (Food allergens once identified can usually be handled by rotation diets in which the substance and other foods in its 'family' are eaten infrequently.) However this may be of only limited value, since it will do little to deal with the underlying immune problem, and may also be difficult to achieve in relation to environmental allergens in the modern world, without virtually withdrawing from it, which is hardly a desirable approach.

Allied to, and often a part of, the problem of allergy and its associated immune dysfunction, is the major problem of toxicity, especially of heavy metals such as lead, cadmium and mercury.

The Mercury Problem

In recent years it has become increasingly obvious that many people have compromised their immune systems through no fault of their own, simply by virtue of the presence in their bodies of mercury which has leached out of the amalgam fillings in their mouth.

Mercury is one of the most toxic substances in existence. For many years amalgams were thought to be stable compounds which, left in the mouth, did no harm. However it has become clear that this is just not true.

An amalgam loses roughly half its mercury content over a very few years and this mercury has to have gone somewhere. Research now shows that it leaves the teeth in several ways. Some leaves as mercury vapour and is absorbed into the saliva and swallowed; some is inhaled into the nasal passages and by diffusion reaches the bloodstream and enters the body this way; some passes along nerve roots serving the teeth and mouth and enters the body (and the brain) in this manner.

Sensitive testing devices can measure the amount of mercury vapour in your mouth before and after you chew, and the rise in such levels is often frighteningly high, especially if there are many fillings in the mouth. Dental experts trying to allay the fears of those pointing to the mercury amalgam danger have stated that the form of the metal used in dentistry, elemental mercury, is not harmful to the body. However it is now known that once in the body, whether absorbed into the digestive system (swallowed with saliva) or inhaled into the lungs or taken in by any other route (skin, nerves etc.), elemental mercury can be changed into the highly toxic methyl mercury by the action of bacteria which live inside all of us.

One of the main reasons for the breakdown of the mercury in amalgam fillings is that the motley selection of metals used together in the mouth can form powerful batteries. Electromotive forces and electrical currents result from the interaction of different metals, with saliva playing the part of a connecting element. Galvanic currents in the mouth have been reported as resulting from dental amalgams since the late nineteenth century and studies of this phenomenon continue to this day (see References), showing a wide range of negative effects, not least the active corrosion of amalgam compounds.

Betsy Russell Manning in her excellent compilation of evidence (*How Safe Are Silver* [mercury] *Fillings?*) states: 'Corrosion of amalgam fillings is well known and well reported, particularly on contact with other compounds (gold, silver). Minute currents and with these electrochemical processes (formation of galvanic elements) will be induced which result in dissolution of amalgams.' Not only toxic (poisoning) effects are then seen but allergic reactions brought about by this toxic irritation, with symptoms as diverse as urticaria and eczema, headaches, asthma and digestive irregularities (colitis etc.).

What Is a Toxic Metal?

Toxic metals can loosely be defined as those which in certain concentrations in the body are known to interfere with normal function. Experience in Japan, in particular with mercury poisoning from contaminated fish (Minimata disease), has shown just what mercury can do to the human body.

The symptoms of mercury toxicity may look familiar to you. They include, at the outset: anxiety, depression, drowsiness, tremors, loss of memory, nervousness.

If mercury toxicity is severe or continues, these early symptoms are followed by: muscle weakness (sometimes progressing to paralysis), numbness and tingling in limbs, visual and speech difficulties, memory loss, loss of co-ordination, emotional instability, etc.

These symptoms when severe are indistinguishable from multiple sclerosis. When mild they match ME perfectly.

Different but equally devastating symptoms can be noted deriving from toxic metal exposure relating to aluminium (aching muscles, senile dementia, liver disorders etc.), copper (arthritis, eczema, anaemia, psychosis etc.), cadmium (fatigue, anaemia, hypertension, kidney and liver problems, etc.) and nickel (breathing problems, anorexia, vomiting, headache etc.). More people are allergic to nickel than all other metals combined, and yet it is used extensively in restorative dentistry.

According to Professor Luid Blanco-Dalmau of the University of Puerto Rico, writing in *The Journal of Prosthetic Dentistry* (vol. 48, no. 1, July 1982), everyone who is having restorative dentistry should be tested for sensitivity to the metals being used by simple patch tests on the skin before they are used. Equipment also exists for rapid screening of the level of mercury vapour being given off inside the mouth.

The ME Connection

If anyone has ME they should think very carefully about the possibility of a heavy metal connection. Was their any dentistry in the year or so prior to the onset of the illness? It does not matter whether this involved new fillings or replacement of old fillings, or the placement of a bridge or crown, or simply a process of scaling and cleaning. All of these procedures could result in the release into the system of toxic metals.

Even if no such procedures were carried out it is possible that a cumulative leaching of mercury and other metals into the system has reached a critical level and that this is adding to the ME problem.

It should be noted that once again, as with candida, it is necessary to forestall criticism by saying that no suggestion is intended that ME and mercury (or other) toxicity are the same thing. However it is clear that, in some instances at least, when the toxicity problem is resolved the underlying symptoms of ME begin to sort themselves out. The presence of heavy metals in the body to any degree is immune suppressing. When they are removed (and they can be) immune activity improves.

Care about Replacement

A veritable industry has arisen around this recent knowledge about amalgam toxicity, with some dentists now spending almost all their time removing amalgams and replacing them with composite (ceramic or plastic) materials or with gold. Care is required before this task is undertaken.

At the outset the electrical potential of all the teeth in the mouth must be measured and recorded. The quadrant (quarter) of the mouth with the lowest electrical potential is then treated first with careful removal of existing fillings and their replacement with safe alternatives. Before these are used they need to be tested to make certain that no new allergic problems are likely.

In the removal of old amalgams strict precautionary procedures must be followed. A rubber dam is placed across the mouth to prevent swallowing of debris and extreme care is exercised to prevent inhalation of powdered debris resulting from drilling. In addition a variety of nutrients which reduce toxic effects of heavy metals are usually supplemented in high dosages at such times. These include calcium and vitamin C as well as amino acids such as cysteine and methionine or the amino acid compound glutathione.

Results and Prospects

Patients previously thought to be suffering from multiple sclerosis have reported miraculous restoration of health after this procedure has been completed. It may take some weeks for benefits to be noted but sometimes they are instantaneous. Many ME patients are also substantially relieved of associated symptoms after amalgam replacement. (See References section for further reading suggestions on this important subject.)

In the spring of 1988 the Swedish government became the first to announce that over the next ten years use of amalgam fillings would be phased out, and that as of the date of the announcement no more fillings of that sort could be used in the teeth of pregnant women. It is to be hoped that other countries will follow the Swedish lead.

Getting Rid of Heavy Metals

Tactics are available for helping to rid the body of toxic metal accumulations. It is also possible by use of hair analysis to test simply for the possibility of such toxicity.

Details of simple self-help measures are given in Chapter 9, which deals with nutritional treatment of ME.

Allergies

Professor James Mowbray is one of the leading medical thinkers who have attempted to engage the ME problem diligently. He has said, 'I have seen very good examples of people who are very well treated by alterations in their environment, i.e. largely the things they were no longer eating, and to define that group [among people with ME] is as important as to define any other group. *The virus group and this group may be entirely separate or they may overlap* [my italics].' (Professor Mowbray classifies one other ME group, who have what he terms 'organic brain disease' such as multiple sclerosis.)

Dr Jonathan Brostoff specializes in the allergy/ME link. He has tried to clarify the overlapping connection between viral activity and allergy in relation to ME. On this subject he says: 'There is no doubt in my clinic that virus infections may bring on, expose, produce or allow to be seen, an ordinary inhalant allergy (and I use allergy in the true sense, e.g. grass, pollen, house dust etc. as an ordinary type of allergy). This is seen in asthmatic children or children with eczema, where the mother will say that her child developed the asthma after a virus infection. It may not have caused it, but the equilibrium may have been moved and the immunity may have become more allergy prone.'

It would once again be fascinating to have recorded just how many children who develop allergic symptoms after a viral 'attack' have been medicated with antibiotics. This is a really vital question, since if a link can be shown, and in many instances it can, then the whole allergy complication becomes clearer, at least to those who accept the candida hypothesis which goes something like this.

Infection (viral or bacterial) leads to antibiotic treatment, which leads to destruction of friendly bacteria, resulting in candida overgrowth and consequent damage to the bowel mucosa by mycelial fungal rhizomes, and therefore undesirable absorption from the gut of wastes, toxins and partially digested food particles with dramatic effects on immune function, resulting in an increase in allergic responses.

Amongst those who support this hypothesis it is usual to treat a child with eczema or asthma by restoring bowel competence (anti-candida programme), thus getting rid of candida overgrowth. The allergic symptoms frequently vanish in the process.

The allergic response to some inhaled substance, such as

pollen or dust, is simply evidence of a vastly hyper-reactive immune function trying to cope with an onslaught of foreign substances entering the body, often from the bowel, due to candida activity. Dr Brostoff deals with the problem by identifying the source of his patients' allergies and then taking them out of contact with these sources, whether food or inhaled substances.

Not all respond, he acknowledges. He also agrees that the cause remains unknown. He does question the role of candida in all this (see his quote in the chapter on candida and ME), and it is to be hoped that the link between these various parts of the puzzle will become clearer to those working in this area of ill-health before too long.

Over the past forty years, according to official government figures, children in the UK have become six times as likely to develop eczema and three times as likely to develop asthma. We might well ask what has happened over this relatively brief time-span to allow such a dramatic decline in immune competence.

Among the various possible causes are three deserving of consideration and investigation. The first is that it was just over forty years ago that antibiotics appeared on the scene. If the candida hypothesis is correct, this alone would account for a greatly increased degree of allergic activity.

Secondly there is the general decline in breast feeding. This leads to very early exposure of the digestive system to foods which the system is often not prepared for. Allergies are commoner in non-breastfed children, and the substances to which they are commonly most allergic are just those very early foods, such as cow's milk products and cereals (with eggs close behind). In studies at Great Ormond Street Hospital in London on children with migraine headaches, asthma, eczema etc. a diet which identifies and then removes common foods such as these usually results in resolution of the problem.

The third and perhaps most controversial possible reason for the explosion of allergic symptoms is that of multiple immunization/vaccination procedures involving 'cocktails' of viral and bacterial substances. It has been suggested by Dr Harold Buttram in the USA that this onslaught, often started in early infancy when the immune system is really very undeveloped, has had a negative overall impact on immune function, despite offering specific protective benefits against certain diseases (although some would doubt the extent of these as well).

This is not the place to expand on these possibilities, but they might produce some thought, especially if the further reading suggestions are followed up. There has to be good reason for the overall decline in immune competence in our children, as evidenced by the terrible statistics relating to increased eczema and asthma. ME and AIDS are just two more examples of a general decline in immune efficiency.

The causes are unlikely to be simple and are probably multiple, with the three elements listed above as a good starting point, followed by the general decline in the health of the planet on which we live. It is hard to imagine that we as dwellers on the earth would not be affected by the pollution of the rivers, seas and atmosphere, the destruction of the life-giving rain forests and the erosion of the protective ozone layer. This is just to give the most obvious examples without specifically looking at the atrocious state of our water supply, contaminated food and electronically and chemically polluted air supply.

In the chapter on 'Lifestyles and ME' a brief look is taken at 'sick building syndrome' which expands somewhat on this last factor of air supply. As these words are being written it is reported that many of the seals of the North Sea are dying from a mysterious viral infection to which they have been made susceptible, it is said, by a decline in their immune function due to contamination of the seas and their food supply.

Similar disasters have been reported on the east coast of America, with dolphins being washed ashore suffering from huge ulcerated lesions and dying of pneumonia. Again, AIDS is given as a comparison. Other fish, too, have had their ecology disrupted and their environment poisoned, with large numbers dying of mysterious viral diseases.

Are we to blame the viruses? Are we to seek vaccines against these? Or are we to try to return the planet to a semblance of health, where the natural immunity of the animals affected, and one hopes of ourselves, would take adequate care of any viruses which might wander by?

Symptoms of Allergy

Allergic symptoms come and go. So do many of the symptoms of ME. It is as well to repeat the statistic uncovered by Dr Patrick Donovan in relation to patients with ME (see Chapter 1). He found that fully 53 per cent of ME patients had a history of allergy.

How many of these were simply suffering from food or substance sensitivity or allergy and nothing more?

The main signs and symptoms which should lead to suspicion of allergy include: fluctuating symptoms; fatigue; mental and psychological problems including depression; fluid retention; weight fluctuations; waking tired after sleep; dark rings under the eyes; muscle and joint pain; racing pulse; low blood sugar with associated dizziness, irritability etc.; digestive symptoms, food cravings or addictions (usually to the food(s) to which you are allergic – alcoholism is an example – see further reading suggestions); headaches and migraines; facial flushing; and of course the obvious allergic symptoms of skin rashes, runny nose or asthma.

How to Deal with Allergies

There are several ways of treating allergy. One is, as we have said, to identity the substance(s) and then to avoid contact.

The identification process is, however, not always easy and a variety of tests are available to help with this, as are methods which involve excluding foods and their families from the diet in order to assess changes in symptoms, followed by reintroduction of foods and careful observation of reactions which follow, if any. Rotation and exclusion diets of this type need to be carefully explained and monitored, ideally by someone familiar with the methods, such as a clinical ecologist or a naturopath.

Short periods of fasting on water only or on very basic foods (pear and lamb diet, 'Stone Age diet') are also methods of noting whether symptoms vanish and then recur as other foods are reintroduced. Again, overall guidance is needed from an expert for best results.

Desensitization of the body by a series of injections of minute quantities of the substance (once it has been identified) is another method of stopping allergic reactions.

Other approaches try generally to detoxify the system (diets, fasts, colonic irrigations) in combination with supplementation of nutrients known to help in such problems (vitamin C, vitamin B5 etc.) as well as use of free-form amino acids to help the body rebuild its defence capabilities.

The scope of this book does not allow for full description of all such methods, and the further reading section is suggested for names of suitable guides to self-help for allergy.

Allergy and the Mind

It is commonly observed that when a person is anxious and stressed their allergy is more pronounced. When the individual is relaxed, allergies seem less reactive. Stephen Davies in the excellent book *Nutritional Medicine*, co-authored with Alan Stewart, says, 'In our experience and that of many other doctors, although it has yet to be proved scientifically, when someone is under emotional or psychological stress, they are more likely to develop a food intolerance . . . In chronic severe food allergies there is often a significant underlying emotional problem.'

It is logical therefore to urge stress reduction and relaxation-type exercises for anyone with allergies, whether, as in ME itself, the allergy results in or is the result of emotional stress.

One snippet of information which defies easy interpretation involves doctors in Boston who were investigating people suffering from the very serious problem of multiple personality syndrome, in which the individual switches without warning from one personality to another. They noted an amazing phenomenon. A patient who was so allergic to cats that she was unable to tolerate them in the room without having a violent asthmatic attack was able to stroke and hold a cat minutes later, after her personality 'switched'. Quite plainly her biochemistry had not altered in this time scale, only her 'mind' control. Yet the allergy was gone, only to return when she reverted to the original personality. What can one make of this? A reading of Dr Paul Pearsall's amazing book *Superimmunity* (see References) will help you to understand the very real links between the mind and allergic responses.

Allergy is often a part of ME, sometimes the major part, sometimes only a side-issue. Toxicity, especially of heavy metals such as mercury, may also be peripheral, or central to, the main problems of ME. Both toxicity and allergy require investigation, and treatment if they are found to be involved. The following strategies should be considered:

1   Have a hair analysis done to look for heavy metal toxicity. This method is widely viewed as effective in detecting toxicity which has occurred during the previous six months or so.
2   If metal toxicity is present, use oral or intravenous chelation methods to assist removal (see Chapter 9).
3   If necessary, see dentist for replacement of amalgams.
4   Consult a clinical ecologist or naturopath in order to assess for dietary and environmental allergens (using rotation and exclusion diets etc., and special tests).
5   Adopt avoidance strategies for known allergens and use an anti-candida type diet (especially acidophilus supplementation) for general and bowel health.
6   Practice stress-reduction and relaxation exercises.

REFERENCES and SUGGESTED FURTHER READING (marked with an *)

How Safe are Silver Fillings? Manning, B. R., Cancer Control Society, Los Angeles 1983.

'Medical Addresses Given at 1985 AGM of UK ME Association', Journal of A NZ ME Society, May 1986.

Multiple Sclerosis: A Self-Help Guide to Its Management, Graham, J., Thorsons, Wellingborough 1987.

Nutritional Influences on Illness, Werbach, M., Third Line Press, Tarzana, California 1987.

Nutritional Medicine, Davies, S., Stewart, A., Pan Books, London 1987.

Superimmunity, Pearsall, P., Ebury Press, London 1987.

Textbook of Natural Medicine (chapters by Buttram on Immunization, and Donovan on Mononucleosis), ed. Pizzorno, J., Murray, M., John Bastyr College Publications, Seattle, Washington 1987.

The Toxic Time Bomb (amalgams), Ziff, S., Thorsons, Wellingborough 1986.
Vaccination and Immunisation: Dangers, Delusions and Alternatives, Chaitow, L., C. W. Daniel, Saffron Walden 1987.

6 The Candida–ME Link

Living inside you, and inside me, are a host of uninvited squatters who have taken up residence in various desirable (for them) parts of the body. One of these is a yeast with a sweet-sounding name but some nasty habits, candida albicans.

Candida is present in every adult and in most children on the planet. It normally does no harm, for it is kept in its place by a variety of other squatters, some of which (unlike candida) perform useful tasks in return for the living accommodation and food which we provide.

Among these are a group of friendly bacteria known as lactobacilli, including acidophilus and bulgaricus (a transient, non-resident friendly bacteria). One of their useful tasks is the production of a B vitamin, biotin, which plays a role in preventing candida from turning into its rampantly aggressive mycelial or fungal form in which it puts down roots (rhizomes) and spreads rapidly.

In its fungal form candida's roots can penetrate the lining of the area in which it normally resides, such as the intestine. When this mucous membrane lining is penetrated by rhizomes it becomes possible for partially digested food particles, toxic wastes, yeast breakdown products etc.

61

to pass through into the bloodstream, resulting in allergies, sensitivities and a constant drain on the immune (defence) mechanisms of the body.

Candida's change from simple yeast to mycelial fungus can be triggered by a variety of events which depress local or general immune function and control of the yeast. Among these is the use of antibiotics in the treatment of infection. Not only are invading, hostile, micro-organisms killed by such drugs but also friendly ones. If this happens to any great degree then a major control of candida is removed.

Other events which can result in yeast overgrowth include use of steroid (hormone-based) drugs such as cortisone and 'the Pill', or other drugs which are immuno-suppressive. Ongoing infection by Epstein-Barr virus or cytomegalovirus can also depress immune function and control of candida. All of these events are encouraged if there happens to be a high level of sugar in the blood (diabetic state or high sugar diet).

A Further Possible Complication

In Chapter 2 which dealt with the virus connection with ME, reference was made to the work of Dr Emanuel Revici, the remarkable nonagenarian who has shown how fungi (e.g. penicillin) can kill and control bacteria and how bacteria can kill and control viruses.

Of course variations also exist in which some yeasts and fungi can be controlled by bacteria (acidophilus controls candida, for example). In general, however, if bacterial presence in an area is severely reduced, as occurs when antibiotics kill off the friendly bacteria in the bowel, this leaves any viral inhabitants free to expand their activity. (Recall also that among the most suspect of all viruses in relation to ME is that family known as enteroviruses, which are inhabitants of the bowel.)

It is often observed, in people with ME, that antibiotics have been used extensively some months prior to the onset of their illness. In some instances, sad to say, antibiotics have been used even though no bacterial infection was current, but 'just in case' such infection developed after or during what was obviously a viral infection.

Now if there was a virus infection, involving enteroviruses, and if antibiotics were given (in the mistaken idea that this was in reality a bacterial infection or 'just in case') there could have been destruction of bacterial control of both candida and enteroviruses, both of which could spread rapidly into regions previously denied them by the now dead 'watchdog' bacteria. It would be of considerable interest to discover just how many people with ME have had antibiotic treatment when it was not absolutely certain that they were bacterially infected.

Symptoms of Candida Overgrowth

Many of the common symptoms seen when yeast overgrowth exists are similar to those of ME. They include fatigue, headaches, depression, sugar craving, digestive complaints, and often a tendency to allergy or food sensitivity, which is probably related to damaged bowel mucosa resulting from rhizome penetration.

One of the simplest ways of proving a connection between ME and candida is to treat the assumed yeast condition and observe the improvement in the symptoms of ME. This may not be 'scientific', but it is usually effective as Sue Finlay can testify.

Sue Finlay's Story

In the *Observer* of 1 June 1986 Sue Finlay told of her battle with ME. She described her decline from an active happy person in her late thirties (some four years prior to the article) into a virtual invalid with a diagnosis of postviral fatigue or ME.

'After an especially bad time – confined to bed, hardly able to stand, tears all day, and suicidal – I decided that rather than wait around indefinitely for the medical scientists to find a solution or for the illness "to burn itself out" I would try to treat the candida and see if things improved.' She persuaded her doctor to give her nystatin, an antifungal drug, and followed general guidelines on candida control given by the New Zealand ME Association which had long recognized this link.

'I began to feel considerably better almost immediately! The feeling of being poisoned left me, a little energy returned, life began to seem a good idea to me. After some months of variable but gradual improvement I came on the book *Candida Albicans – Could Yeast Be Your Problem?* by Leon Chaitow. I changed my diet radically. I cut out all sugars and refined carbohydrates. All bread, mushrooms, tea, alcohol, vinegar, coffee and chocolate were dropped. All these foods feed the yeast. I used vitamin supplements to enhance the immune system, olive oil and garlic to attack the yeast and acidophilus powder to replace the candida with healthy intestinal flora. I ate vegetables, salads, whole cereals and fruit in abundance. At present I am able to walk nearly half a mile without total collapse, I am beginning to work in the garden a little. I still have to rest every day and be very careful not to overdo things and cause a relapse, but I have had eight months of improvement and am steadily reducing the nystatin.'

Some months after this article appeared Sue Finlay wrote to me as follows: 'I've now been eleven months on nystatin and about six months on "your" regime. I have been able to leave off nystatin for a month and feel good. Not "sick", until I over-exert myself when I do get exhausted, sore and stroppy/weepy. But my abilities are greatly improved on last year when I was a gibbering wreck unable to walk 25 yards. I can walk half-a-mile, mow the grass, cope fairly adequately with far more visitors and get through the day if I have a rest after lunch. It's great to have this much restored to me. *I feel the candida is under control but the underlying problem remains. Now to tackle it* [my italics].'

ME Is Not Candida

This last sentence is really very important. There is not meant to be any suggestion that the symptoms and condition of ME is all down to candida.

But it is observable, and Sue Finlay's story is but one of hundreds, that if the candida problem is dealt with matters often improve to the point where the person afflicted is capable of doing something constructive about the underlying problems of immune deficiency, allergy, nutritional deficiencies, possible heavy metal toxicity, hyperventilation, or whatever else is operating along with possible persistent viral activity.

Sue Finlay's Strategy

The brief outline which Sue Finlay gave of her regime when she undertook an anti-candida programme requires some elaboration.

She correctly identifies refined carbohydrates and sugars as 'feeding' the yeast. Any home wine-maker will know that yeasts of all sorts love sugar. If the system is deprived (as far as it is possible) of sugar in concentrated or refined forms, from food sources, this slows down candida activity.

The other foods mentioned by her, chocolate, tea, coffee, vinegar, mushrooms etc. are not foods which feed yeast (except for their sugar content) but rather they are all high in mould (e.g. on tea) or are derived from fermentation processes which involve yeast. Because of the damage to the bowel mucosa and the spread of candida, the body becomes sensitized to yeasts and is more likely to react in an allergic manner to any substances derived from or containing these (moulds, spores etc.).

For this reason in the first months of an anti-candida diet any food or drink which has involved fermentation or yeast in its production, or which is likely to have mould (old nuts, dried fruit etc.) on it should be avoided.

A variety of antifungal substances are also incorporated into the programme including olive oil (for its oleic acid) and garlic, both of which retard or destroy candida. A derivative of coconuts, caprylic acid, is used as a fungus killer in preference to nystatin because the latter is itself yeast-based and research at the Washington University School of Medicine shows that ultimately when nystatin is stopped it often results in even more colonies of yeast than were present before its use. Caprylic acid (caprycin) has no such rebound effect when its use ceases after candida is controlled (we never actually get rid of it, only try to get it back under control).

In addition, acidophilus and other cultures are taken to repopulate the bowel and this is a most important part of the strategy. Biotin, which controls the change in the yeast to its fungal form, is also supplemented. (A brief outline of the anti-candida programme is given in Chapter 9.)

Doctors Differ in Their Attitude to Candida

There are mixed views expressed by doctors working with ME as far as candida is concerned. Dr Jonathan Brostoff is on record as saying, '. . . I don't think it is clear from anybody's work yet what role candida plays in the whole syndrome. . . . We may be seeing [in candida overgrowth] a disease which is only twenty, forty or fifty years old which is a direct result of antibiotic treatment. We have had a number of patients who have not responded to chemical avoidance, food, nutrition or whatever, but seem to have responded to the treatment of putative [assumed] over-growth of candida in the gut. That is just treating candida with nystatin and a low-carbohydrate diet. We presume the nystatin only works on the candida and therefore presume that lowering the candida in the gut has helped, but there is no direct evidence.'

Whilst this may not strictly amount to 'direct evidence', it could, nevertheless, be argued that the evidence is strongly indicative.

In the ME Association's Summer 1988 Newsletter Dr David Smith says: 'Candida is a yeast that is commensal in the human body. This means that it can be found on most of the surfaces of the body and surfaces here also include the openings of the body and tubes in between connected to those openings . . . It is your body's innate natural defence mechanisms that keep the various bacteria and yeasts under control. Candida is also kept under control by other bacteria that live on the skin or in these various places . . . If you do something or take something or have something which lowers this localized resistance to candida then the candida, instead of being a harmless spore on your skin or in your mouth, will kill the localized bacteria or inhibit your immune system generally.'

Dr Smith continues: 'Antibiotics can kill off localized bacteria, and thrush [candida] takes over. A lot of anti-biotics like broad-spectrum ampicillin kill the bacteria not only in the mouth and the gut but also in the vagina, and a superimposed candida infection often occurs.' But he goes on to say, 'I am not aware of this type of infection having any systemic action, and whether people with chronic infection of the mouth or the vagina due to thrush have any significant systemic illness I do not know, but I do not believe so.'

Having acknowledged that candida can systematically invade an individual who is severely immune compromised, or who had excessive antibiotics, he then states, 'I appreciate that the prolonged use of antibiotics, the contraceptive pill etc. can cause candida problems but as far as I am aware they are not associated with ME. Whether or not people with ME get a lot of antibiotics at the beginning is immaterial. I cannot see that there is any evidence that these types of problems are associated with candida.'

The fact is, however, that candida has a virulent fungal form and that the damage this form is able to inflict can greatly complicate the picture, bringing about a variety of systemic problems, including the further compromising of immune function and multiple allergies. It is not easy to agree that past antibiotic treatment of people with ME, and possible candida involvement, is necessarily immaterial to their condition.

On the other hand, Dr Celia Wookey, already mentioned in Chapter 2 and herself a sufferer from ME, wrote in the *Daily Telegraph* (19 July 1988) as follows: 'One area crying out for good scientific investigation is the link between allergy and candida. ME depresses the immune system, so that candida infections are probably more common than realized. One encouraging sign is that some hospitals are now carrying out blood tests for candida antibodies. There is also increasing interest in how ME patients may be helped through treatment of food allergies.'

Dr Wookey is looking for the candida/allergy link and seems to assume that candida overgrowth results from ME's depressing effect on the immune system. It might equally be argued, however, that the candida overgrowth came first, depressed the immune system, and allowed the viral activity which led to ME.

This latter sequence seems at least to be likely in many of the cases I have treated. It is also the opinion apparently of Dr Belinda Dawes. She is quoted in *Cosmopolitan* (February 1988) as holding the view that ME is due to weakness of the immune system brought on by an infestation of the gut by naturally occurring yeast (candida) which gets out of control.

Dr Dawes has cured herself and many patients with ME using a nutritional approach and, according to *Cosmopolitan*, claims that 75 per cent of ME patients can be helped in this way (diet and vitamins, stimulation of immune function, anti-allergy, anti-candida), although this can take several years to achieve.

Have You a Candida Overgrowth?

Dr Wookey speaks of hospitals now testing for yeast antibodies. Is this the way to know whether or not candida is active?

Regrettably such tests are not entirely accurate. We all have candida in and on us. The likelihood is that in most people some degree of antibody activity is present (this indicates that the immune system has defended itself against the yeast). However if immune function is weak, such a response may not be forthcoming and a test could show little or no antibody presence while active candida yeast overgrowth was continuing.

A far more reliable method of identifying candida activity is to look at your history and your symptoms. This can point quite accurately to a current candida overgrowth. The following are the major associated symptoms. They are more likely to be active if one or more of the following events has been true for you:

1   A course of antibiotics for eight weeks or longer or for a number of shorter periods four or more times in one year.

2 Antibiotic treatment for acne for a month or more.
3 A course of cortisone, prednisone or ACTH (steroid treatment).
4 The use of contraceptive medication (the Pill) for a year or more.
5 Treatment with immunosuppressive drugs.
6 More than one pregnancy.

The major symptom picture of active candida includes at least some of the following. If two or more of these symptoms is common or current, and one or more of the list above is true for you, then candida is probably a current problem in your life, requiring specific action (see Chapter 9).

- Recurrent or persistent cystitis, prostatitis or vaginitis.
- Endometriosis.
- Thrush (oral, or vaginal) more than once.
- Athlete's foot, fungal nail or skin infection.
- Extreme sensitivity to chemical fumes, perfumes, tobacco smoke.
- You feel worse after eating yeasty or sugary foods or drinks.
- Allergic symptoms.
- Abdominal bloating, distension, diarrhoea or constipation.
- Premenstrual syndrome (fluid retention, irritability etc.).
- Depression, fatigue, lethargy, poor memory, inability to concentrate.
- Muscular aches for no obvious reason, tingling, numbness etc.
- Swollen or aching joints for no obvious reason.
- Vaginal discharge, irritation. Menstrual cramps or pain.
- Impotence or loss of sexual desire.

- Erratic vision; spots before the eyes.

This list of candida-related symptoms clearly overlaps with the symptoms of ME and it is not easy always to decide the origin of such problems. The majority of ME patients with candida will find that not only one or two of the list applies to them but usually more than half of it. In that case I would urge you to approach the candida overgrowth aspect of the problem as being most likely to respond rapidly to self-help measures.

REFERENCES

'All in the Mind – or in the Body Too?' Wookey, C., *Daily Telegraph*, 19 July 1988, p. 13.

'An Illness Doctors Don't Recognise', Finlay, S., *Observer*, 1 June 1986, p. 43.

Candida Albicans: Could Yeast Be Your Problem? Chaitow, L., Thorsons, Wellingborough 1985.

'Chronic Mononucleosis-Like Syndrome', Donovan, P., in *Textbook of Natural Medicine* (Pizzorno and Murray eds), JBCNM, Seattle 1987.

'Dear Dr Smith', *Journal of ME Association*, Summer 1988, p. 6.

'Medical Addresses at 1985 AGM ME Association of UK', Journal of ANZ ME Society, May 1986, p. 48.

'ME and You', Holmes, P., *Cosmopolitan*, February 1988, pp. 91–4.

The Missing Diagnosis (Chronic Candidiasis), Truss, C. O., MD, published by the author, 2614 Highland Avenue, Birmingham, Alabama 35205, 1982.

The Yeast Connection, Crook, W., PO Box 3494, Jackson, Tennessee 38301, 1983.

7 Nutrition as Immune Enhancer and Immune Suppressor

Your daily eating habits have a profound effect on the efficiency, or otherwise, of your immune system.

If you have health problems involving allergy or candida overgrowth then you will already be well aware of the connection between what you eat and how well, or ill, you feel.

If you have no such problems but do have ME then the relationship between your dietary habits and your state of health is going to be equally important, and what you eat (and probably what you supplement) will almost certainly have a profound effect on the rate and nature of your recovery.

Many of the daily foods and non-foods which are consumed are immune-suppressing, and these need to be eliminated from your diet, as far as is possible. Other foods, because of their nutrient content, are immune-enhancing, and these need to be included as a regular part of your daily dietary pattern. I will give lists of such foods (good and bad) later in this chapter.

Supplementation – Why Is It Necessary?

In addition to the foods you eat it is usually necessary to suggest additional supplementation of some (sometimes many) of the nutrients they contain. This is because of known immune-enhancing functions which many of these possess, as well as to match greatly increased demands which the body has for certain nutrients when you are under stress or when infection is current or recently past.

It is now known, beyond doubt, thanks to the research work of the late Professor Roger Williams of Texas University, that we all have variable requirements for particular nutritional elements. In any group of people there is a demonstrable variation of the actual biochemical *need* for particular nutrients such as the individual vitamins, minerals and trace elements. This variation in biological/physiological need can be as much as 700 per cent between individuals for some nutrients.

These needs are to a large extent genetically programmed, inborn, unchangeable. Thus you may need four, five or seven times more vitamin C than I do, in order to function at your optimum level of health, and in turn you may require half the calcium that I require. And so on through a list of nearly fifty nutrients without which neither you nor I could survive for long in good health.

Needs Change

In addition to such inherited biochemical individuality there are very many circumstances in which nutritional requirements alter. In infancy, childhood and puberty, and especially as we grow older, there are special requirements for some nutrients to meet the patterns of growth and change under way.

During illness, pregnancy, lactation, periods of stress, at

73

the menopause, during infection, when exposed to pollution, and when extra exercise is taken, you and I, and everyone else, will need additional nutrient intake to meet the requirements of the body.

In old age special needs exist to compensate for the poor digestive, absorption and assimilative functions which are so common, and it has been shown that nutritional supplementation of the elderly increases cellular immune function which is primarily involved in surveillance and regulation of viral infections.

When a condition such as ME is current, specific additional nutrient needs are certain, and many of these can be met by supplementation.

Can Nutritional Needs Not Be Met from the Diet Alone?

Possibly, under ideal conditions, the diet could provide all the required nutrients, even those heroically required to meet inherited or acquired needs.

However ideal conditions seldom prevail in modern industrial settings, as far as food is concerned. Such factors as commercial food production methods; lengthy gaps between harvesting, marketing and eventual consumption; dubious preparation methods; and the unknown quantity of just what foods are selected, all add up to a situation in which the probability of a wholly adequate diet becomes doubtful.

In addition the likelihood is that, if you have ME, your digestive capabilities, not to mention the functions of absorption and utilization of nutrients, may well be impaired to some extent. What enters your mouth in the food you eat may therefore not be 'bio-available' for your body cells because of all or any of the factors mentioned.

Supplementation of nutrients, known to be required for

function as well as for healing, is therefore a method of assuring that at least basic requirements are met.

Patrick Donovan in his chapter on 'Chronic Mononucleosis-Like Syndrome' (Epstein-Barr infection) in the *Textbook of Natural Medicine* states, in relation to the treatment of viral infection: 'A basic high-quality multi-vitamin and mineral supplement high in B complex vitamins (especially B6, B12, folate and pantothenic acid) and trace minerals (particularly zinc, selenium, chromium and manganese) is an essential supplement baseline. In addition three specific nutrients should be emphasized for their immune-enhancing activity.'

These three nutrients are the carotenes (found in plant foods) which are made into vitamin A by the body, vitamin C which is known to have antiviral properties, and zinc which is vital for the effective function of the thymus gland, the very heart of the immune system.

Research by Professor Emanuel Cheraskin in the United States (discussed in his co-authored book *Diet and Disease*, 1977) has shown that in modern industrialized cities, when thousands of apparently healthy individuals from all social and economic classes were examined, *over 80 per cent showed themselves to be deficient in at least one of the major nutrient factors (vitamin, mineral)* as determined by official recommended levels. Over 60 per cent showed deficiencies of two or more nutrient factors. These were ostensibly healthy individuals. What of people not even outwardly healthy?

A prudent and realistic approach to regaining competent immune function, and with it renewed energy, requires the use of concentrated, easily absorbed nutrients. These can be seen as the raw materials from which the organs, systems, biochemical pathways and functions of the body can derive their essential specifically needed elements and substances.

New Zealand Study of ME and Diet

A nutritionist and an osteopath in New Zealand (which has a disproportionately high incidence of ME) combined their efforts in a study of the effectiveness of a programme to help ME.

Warren Stewart and Chris Rowe state, 'Doing *one* thing to correct the condition (of ME) is obviously not enough. What is called for is a major influence on body function by a powerful supplementation programme aimed at facilitating immune system function, helping fat metabolism, improving digestion and alleviating fatigue.' They reasoned that:

1   Digestion would be improved by supplementation of enzymes which aid digestive function. This would reduce the possibility of partially digested fragments being absorbed through the compromised bowel mucus membrane as well as reducing the food supply for candida.
2   Bowel function would be improved, resulting in fewer toxic residues being absorbed, thus also giving less opportunity for candida to proliferate further.
3   Fat digestion would be enhanced if bile salts were supplemented.
4   Fatigue would be reduced if nutrient support were given to the adrenal gland (based on results of previous animal studies).
5   Nutritional enhancement of the immune system would speed overall healing.

Two small groups of ME patients (12 people in all, diagnosed both by their own doctors and the researchers as having ME) were assembled. They were asked to record daily, for the next seven weeks, a number of indicators as to their condition such as tiredness on waking, feelings of 'wellness', bowel and digestive status, work-output levels, degree of muscle/joint pain or ache and so on.

During the first week no supplementation was allowed in order to establish a 'base-line' for these various self-observed indicators. In subsequent weeks one group received a number of nutrient supplements including digestive enzymes and immune-enhancing substances. The other group (the control or 'placebo' group) received dummy nutrients of the same size, smell and colour containing inert, non-allergenic substances. The researchers were unaware, during the study, which group was receiving real, and which dummy, substances.

After three weeks the supplementation pattern was switched so that those previously receiving dummy tablets started getting 'the real thing' and vice versa.

At the end of the study the participants were asked to continue keeping their daily recording of indicators in a diary. Only two patients failed to show positive improvement; one of these was noted to be under considerable emotional stress and the other had a far wider range of symptoms as compared with the others in the study. Of the 12 starting the trial 10 completed it.

Statistical analysis of such a small group is not of course conclusive. However it was established that, in general, of the seven patients who improved in energy terms there was an approximately 33 per cent increase on average (ranging from 11 to 66 per cent). Digestive function improved in eight of those supplemented, by an average of 35 per cent (with a range of 11 to 65 per cent).

The variations seen during the various stages of the study (receiving no supplements, real supplements or dummy supplements) tended to confirm that these were playing a major part in the altered energy and digestive levels recorded. When digestive enzymes were supplemented a noticeable improvement occurred in digestive function of those (the majority) who improved. When this happened energy levels also increased. The converse was also seen –

when digestion became more troublesome, so did energy levels decrease even further.

The researchers observe that a problem in working with people with ME is that their condition reduces their motivation and ability to co-operate. A further observation is that, against all advice, when a modicum of energy returned, they tended to do too much or failed to stay as closely as they had previously to their assigned dietary patterns.

The conclusions of the researchers is of interest. Having observed that the experimental supplementation appeared to provide the basis for improvement in most of those participating, they state: 'Other physical and psychological problems need to be attended to as well as a considerably longer term of taking supplements than was feasible in this study. It is also apparent that a supplementation programme needs to be tailored to each individual, changing as the condition changes.' This would seem to be the ideal.

Supplementation cannot cure ME. It can, however, support and assist the recovery of the person with ME, if it is designed to meet particular needs and if other elements of the condition are simultaneously dealt with.

Experience of Other Doctors Supports New Zealand Results

Dr Belinda Dawes, mentioned earlier, who treats ME and has the disease herself, is reported as claiming that she can help 75 per cent of ME patients, using a combination of dietary changes and nutritional supplementation as well as anti-candida and anti-allergy approaches. It can, she says, take as long as several years for full results to be felt.

In Chapter 9 I will detail the supplements most usually found to help in ME. Some of these are immune-enhancing, others relate to anti-candida and antiviral properties, while others are energy-enhancing nutrients such as germanium and coenzyme-Q_{10}, or relate to avoidance of a low-blood sugar level for which chromium (part of the glucose tolerance factor) may be supplemented.

Other Nutritional Influences

Certain nutritional tactics have been shown to have specific effects on viral activity, at least in relation to some viruses.

Herpes simplex causes unpleasant and debilitating crops of vesicles on the face or the genitalia. It has been known for some years that certain foods appear to affect the condition when it is active. Those foods rich in the amino acid lysine (fish, chicken, beans, eggs, potatoes etc.) seem to help in moderating and soothing the problem, allowing for rapid healing, whereas foods rich in another amino acid, arginine (chocolate, peanuts, nuts, seeds, cereals), seem to do the opposite, delaying healing and aggravating the lesions. Lysine supplementation is also used successfully in this way.

Lysine and arginine are similar chemically, and it is believed that the virus, which replicates more quickly in the presence of arginine, may be 'fooled' into utilizing lysine instead, with less satisfactory results for itself but better ones for the unfortunate host to all this activity.

It has been shown by research that when we are stressed the relative levels of lysine and arginine circulating in the bloodstream alter, towards a higher arginine level. Even the mild stress of sunburn is seen to result in this change. Anyone with herpes will know that lying in the sun is an excellent method of reactivating the dormant virus and producing an attack of vesicles.

Once again we can see just how nutritional and stress-related factors interact, and how one can influence the other. If, in the case of herpes, stress (sunburn or anything else) tilts the lysine-arginine ratio towards a more favourable situation for the virus it is possible to tilt it back to a more protective ratio nutritionally.

It would of course be ideal for both the mental/emotional and the nutritional elements to be working together in this direction, and this is the theme I wish to impress on anyone with ME. No single approach is likely to be rapidly successful in your condition. Use of all those elements which are mutually supportive of healing is the ideal.

It is often possible that in any particular case of ME there is an element of persistent viral activity (not herpes but perhaps Coxsackie-B) and that similar nutritional (and stress-reducing) tactics may apply.

Food and Immune Function

Studies in humans (there are numerous animal studies but these are not always relevant to humans) show the following effects on specific aspects of immune function as a result of nutritional imbalance. (Note: in looking at these, remember that Professor Cheraskin has observed that at least 80 per cent of normal healthy adults are deficient in one or more of the major nutrients).

1 The function of the lymphatic system and the presence of lymphocytes in the blood are depressed by deficiency of vitamin B6, iron or zinc.
2 The ratio between the all-important T- and B-cells is altered negatively by deficiency of vitamin A, folic acid (a B vitamin) or iron.
3 The so-called proliferative response, or defence action of the lymphocytes, against infection is reduced by deficiency of vitamin B12, folic acid, iron and zinc, and by too much vitamin E and essential fatty acids.
4 The immunoglobulin response is negatively affected

80

by deficiency of pantothenic acid (vitamin B5) and vitamin B6.

5   Overall resistance is reduced by deficiency of vitamin A, thiamin (B1), folic acid, vitamin D, iron and zinc, and by excessive amounts of iron.

6   Antibody production is depressed if vitamin B2 (riboflavin) or magnesium or selenium are deficient.

7   Supplementation with any of these as needed (according to deficiency indications) or of amino acids such as taurine, glutamine and of full-spectrum free-form amino acids (see below) enhances immune function.

Greater insight into the complexity of the relationship between the immune system and nutrition will be gained by reading Professor Melvyn Werbach's excellent summary of this in the chapter 'Immunodepression' in his book *Nutritional Influences on Illness* as well as Dr Michael Weiner's *Maximum Immunity*, and the brilliant book *Superimmunity* by Dr Paul Pearsall.

Protein. Adequate protein is vital for proper immune function, and its deficiency results in a multiple compromising of aspects of defence and recovery. In the case of people with impaired digestive function it is suggested that the amino acids which together make up protein be provided in supplement form in order to assure their presence in the body in a 'free' form, as though already digested.

Full-spectrum, free-form amino acids are available from many reputable suppliers, and depending upon the degree of digestive impairment can be safely supplemented on a daily basis to ensure that optimum protein levels are present for repair, regeneration and energy production.

Sugar. The negative aspects of sugar consumption in relation to their effects on candida have already been discussed (Chapter 6), but it is not generally realized that consumption of sugar in its refined form has a specific immune-depressing effect. Studies show that as much as a 50 per cent drop in what is called neutrophil phagocytosis occurs after an intake of 75 grams of sugar (sucrose, fructose, glucose, honey, fruit juice all had the same effect) within 30 minutes of consumption and lasting for up to five hours, with the peak of depressed activity two hours after ingestion. These neutrophils constitute fully 70 per cent of the white blood cell population and such depression represents a major compromising of the defence capability of the body. If infection is present, as it is in many instances of ME, such a reduction in surveillance potential is critically important.

Sugar consumption also aggravates a condition of low blood sugar (hypoglycaemia) which is discussed below.

Sugar, any colour, any type, should be reduced to nil for anyone with ME. Refined flour products do not have the same direct effect on immune function, but since they are made up of many 'empty calories', containing as they do little of nutritional value, they are undesirable in an ME patient's diet in anything but minute amounts.

Fats. Immune function is reduced by the additional load of excessive cholesterol, triglycerides and other fat-related fractions in the blood. A low-fat diet is called for, together with a high intake of complex carbohydrates such as whole grains, fruits and vegetables and of course pulses, nuts and seeds (these contain multiple vitamin, mineral and trace element constituents as well as fibre which reduces fat levels). This particular aspect of nutritional imbalance can be aided further by use of the amino acid carnitine which assists in the reduction of fat-related substances from the bloodstream.

Digestive aids. If, as is generally the case, digestive function has been impaired in anyone with ME, certain strategies need to be adopted to assist a return to some degree of normality. These will be discussed in Chapter 9 which outlines the ideal diet as well as the supplements probably required for people with ME. Improved digestive function may require additional digestive acids, digestive enzymes, natural laxatives, bowel flora support from additional lactobacilli ('friendly' bacteria) or from herbal products which improve certain aspects of digestion or elimination, or all of these.

Food, Energy and Some Nasty By-Products

Since one of the major elements of ME is lack of energy, it is of some importance that we look at energy production in the body.

At its simplest, food nutrients and oxygen are transported to the cells of the body by the blood. They enter the cell where minute 'factories' called mitochondria carry out energy production. An 'energy molecule' known as ATP (adenosine triphosphate) is formed from the oxygen and the food (as are some highly undesirable by-products called free radicals) and it is then transported to wherever it is needed to be used in mechanical, chemical, electrical or other work functions. Energy production is enhanced by the use of specific nutrients such as germanium and coenzyme Q_{10}. The recommended levels of supplementation will be given in Chapter 9.

The waste products of the initial energy production, the free radicals, are of some considerable importance since these highly charged particles are capable, unless rapidly deactivated by the body, of doing serious cellular damage. They can destroy cell walls or react with other substances to form highly toxic elements in the body. Free radicals are considered to be the cause of some cancers, arthritic changes, circulatory and cardiac problems due to damage induced in arterial walls, and much more.

In good health we have an abundance of free radical scavengers and quenchers which are capable of deactivating and making safe these anarchic sub-molecular hooligans. Unfortunately in poor health such defensive activity declines.

The commonest of the free radicals associated with energy production are known as superoxide and hydrogen peroxide (bleach). When these meet they form an even more powerful radical called hydroxyl. Together these cause an enormous amount of cellular damage and are largely responsible for many diseases and for the more obvious signs of ageing such as wrinkles, stiffness and reduced functional ability in tissues.

The protection against these comes from specific antagonists to the radicals. These are enzymes such as superoxide dismutase (deactivates superoxide) and catalase (deactivates hydrogen peroxide) as well as gluta-thione peroxidase and methionine reductase.

These enzymes are supported in their protective role against free radicals by antioxidant nutrients such as vitamin A (or its precursor beta carotene), vitamin C, vitamin E and selenium. They (the enzyme free radical scavengers) are now known to be capable of direct supplementation after recent studies in Mexico which show increased blood levels after the taking by mouth of enzyme-rich substances derived from freshly sprouted wheat (fresh seedlings and sprouts are very rich in these protective enzymes). It is also possible to increase their levels by supplementation of their mineral precursors such as selenium and zinc.

What Has This to Do with ME?

All cases of chronic ill-health, all cases of immune depression, all cases of nutritional imbalance (and ME usually involves some or all of these) result in depressed enzyme activity and increased free radical activity. This may relate directly to symptoms such as allergy, inflammation, pain and stiffness.

Direct supplementation of the raw materials from which the body manufactures its own enzyme protectors and energy cycle agents, as well as of enzymes themselves, is a powerful means of reducing this burden of free radical activity and restoring normality out of chaos.

The Hypoglycaemia Connection

When you eat food which contains sugar (an apple, wholemeal flour) but which itself is intact (not juiced or refined) the sugar in it is *slowly* absorbed into the body as digestion releases it from its associated food substances. This results in a gentle rise in blood sugar levels which is easily controlled by the body's balancing mechanism for this (storage of any sugar above normal requirements or its deactivation by the release of a small amount of insulin from its production site, the pancreas).

If, however, the food is processed – say the wheat is refined (made into white flour by removal of the outer layer) or in the case of the apple, juiced – the sugars become much more easily absorbed (in the case of the juice this is almost instantaneous) and a *rapid* rise in blood sugar takes place. This is less easily dealt with, and a correspondingly rapid release of insulin is called for to normalize the now-high sugar levels. If the diet contains multiple intakes of refined sugary foods and sugared drinks this pattern repeats frequently.

Recall that a condition of permanent high blood sugar is the diabetic state and that this leads to massive tissue damage, cardiac problems etc. It is essential for the body to maintain levels of sugar in the blood at the correct level and not to allow the level to increase above an optimum point for too long.

If stimulants such as tea, coffee (sugared or otherwise) or other caffeine-containing substances such as chocolate or cola are consumed, or if tobacco or alcohol are used, the adrenal glands are stimulated to produce adrenalin which gives the person a 'lift' (the usual reason for taking these substances) and simultaneously releases into the bloodstream stored sugar. If this is not needed for immediate energy utilization it has to be dealt with by the pancreas and its insulin production, just as in the fruit juice and refined flour example above.

If anxiety is present or if there are repetitive instances of stress and reaction to events, the 'fight or flight' mechanism of the body which prepares it for activity in the face of a perceived threat operates, and again causes the adrenals to release adrenalin, increase blood sugar levels etc., etc.

Here, then, is a picture of modern homo sapiens. Stressed and anxious, consuming nutritionally bankrupt, sugar-rich food, and using stimulants many times each day. Sugar floods the system in response to all of these insults and the pancreas works overtime to maintain a semblance of balance.

The Result

In the end the efficiency of the pancreas in its response to these demands may become impaired. What usually happens, it is thought by many experts, is that after a while – as stress and stimulants increase their demands on the progressively weaker adrenals – the pancreas over-responds, producing too much insulin and therefore a depression of blood sugar below what is normal.

This makes the person involved feel shaky, anxious,

lightheaded, forgetful, nervous, fatigued etc., etc., and usually produces an immediate craving for something sweet or a stimulant (yet another cigarette, alcoholic drink or cup of coffee) in order to get the sugar levels up, with associated relief from the symptoms of low blood sugar (hypoglycaemia).

And so the merry-go-round progresses. Somewhere in all this many ME patients will see echoes of their former existence and recognize some of the seeds which grew into their present condition.

How to Recognize Hypoglycaemia in Yourself

If you tend to wake up feeling tired, if as mealtimes approach you feel lightheaded, irritable and shaky, if you feel far more energetic after eating and often find yourself craving sweet foods or wishing strongly for a stimulant such as tea or coffee (especially between meals), and if when you miss a meal or a between meal snack you feel really unwell, then hypoglycaemia is almost certainly part of your problem. This is not true of all or even the majority of people with ME, in my experience. But it is true of some.

In this whole sorry mess there is a further complication which may emerge. As the adrenals and the pancreas (which not only produces insulin, remember, but also protein-digesting enzymes) become ever more exhausted, allergic reactions may become part of the picture. This further compromises the immune system.

Addiction to, or dependence upon, substances associated with the cravings involved in boosting sugar levels or masking the allergic response, may become fixed. Thus anyone who craves a particular food (or class of foods) is probably allergic to it and may be addicted to it.

The fatigue element of hypoglycaemia may or may not be part of the picture in anyone with ME. If it is, it calls for some specific supplementation (chromium for example) as well as a dietary strategy of eating little and often, combined with avoidance of stimulants, avoidance of sugar-rich or refined foods, and reduction in stress and arousal levels. Some guidelines will be given in Chapter 9.

Whether we are trying to reduce candida or viral activity, or to enhance a depressed immune system, or to deal with the complications of previous habits which have resulted in allergy or hypoglycaemia, nutrition is a major element in recovery of health for the person with ME. Both a balanced and ordered dietary pattern as well as (in almost all cases) supplementation of nutrients can help in some or all of the interlocking areas of this puzzling (but all things considered, not surprising) syndrome.

REFERENCES

The Beat-Fatigue Workbook, Chaitow, L., Thorsons, Wellingborough 1988.
Diet and Disease, Cheraskin, E., Ringstoef, W., Clark, J., Keats, New Canaan 1977.
Low Blood Sugar (Hypoglycaemia): The 20th Century Epidemic, Budd, M., Thorsons, Wellingborough 1986.
Maximum Immunity, Weiner, M., Gateway Books, Bath 1987.
Nutritional Influences on Illness, Werbach, M., Third Line Press, Tarzana, California 1987, and Thorsons 1989.
Superimmunity, Pearsall, P., Ebury Press, London 1987.
Textbook of Natural Medicine, Pizzorno, J., Murray, M., JBCNM, Seattle 1987.

8 ME, Sleep, Exercise, Environment and Lifestyle

Other than what we eat, and how we react to the stresses of life including toxic and infectious assaults which assail our systems, there are habitual and environmental factors which deserve attention in so far as they may contribute to or encourage the symptoms of ME.

The Story So Far

We may be born with certain idiosyncratic nutritional requirements which are unlikely to be met by the foods we choose to eat in our daily lives. Genetically we may also be predisposed to certain health problems (such as allergy) which make ME more likely by weakening the immune system. Genetically acquired tendencies or early training may, in addition, 'programme' us towards unsatisfactory patterns of behaviour or to poor stress-coping abilities which lead to a further reduction in the effectiveness of our defence systems.

We may further add to such disadvantages by eating and drinking in such a way as to deplete our immune systems even more, either through under-consumption (deficiencies) or over-consumption of undesirable foods (sugars, fats etc.), both of which extremes negatively influence immune function as we have seen in the previous chapter.

This general decline in health status can be made infinitely more serious and complex by the addition of toxicities resulting from the acquisition of chemicals (pesticides, fungicides etc.) or such heavy metals as lead and mercury, to which we are all increasingly exposed from a multitude of possible sources, including our food, the atmosphere and even from dental work (see Chapter 5 on toxicity and allergy).

All or any of the above can lead to a chronically toxic state of affairs in the body in general and the bowel in particular, where the ecology may become disturbed, resulting in yeast, viral, bacterial or protozoal infections.

After the initial, short-term, benefits of drugs, such as antibiotics, used in response to these and other infections, the situation in the bowel often worsens due to local antibiotic-induced ecological disasters involving the destruction of friendly bacteria, followed by chronic bowel toxicity and rampant yeast (candida) spread. Allergies, deficiencies and toxicities then become worse still.

If habitually there is also the (ab)use of stimulants (tea, coffee, alcohol, cigarettes etc.) then further problems may develop involving blood sugar levels, adrenal and pancreatic exhaustion, with consequent decline in the overall functioning of the body. Further complications in the internal balance of the body may result from use of prescribed or 'social' drugs, including 'the Pill'.

A viral (or any other) infection occurring in anyone thus compromised would find a fine soil in which to grow, coupled with a weak defence to overcome. Associated with this sad but not uncommon series of events, and accompanying the general decline in health towards what Professor Jeffrey Bland has called a state of being 'vertically ill' (as opposed to horizontally ill when we actually take to our bed), it may be anticipated that a degree of depression would be present. This makes immune function even weaker. A chronic infection, such as often exists in ME, could well be the result.

Do we really dare to anticipate a simple, 'magic-bullet', cure for anyone who is ill in this way, as a result of such a complex series of unconnected yet interrelated causes? Is it likely that dealing with any single element in this maze of problems will normalize the situation?

Is it not more likely that the elements which have battered the body into a state in which it can no longer function normally, never mind defend itself from further attacks and onslaughts, all require attention, removal or resolution, before 'cure' of the multitude of possible symptoms which may be present, currently or intermittently, can be expected?

We have in earlier chapters briefly surveyed many of the possible elements which can lead to the all-too-common pattern of 'burn-out' which I have described in the previous few paragraphs. And there are others also in need of at least a mention, lest we overlook their importance.

The number of hours set aside for exercise and sleep are important elements in the continuing well-being of the human organism, and both of these are of some importance in recovery from ME.

Exercise

Anyone with ME must not introduce active physical exercise into their programme of recovery or maintenance until they are well on the way to restoring health, for their muscles just cannot be exercised without aggravating the symptoms.

However, ultimately, physical recovery does involve the

reintroduction of exercise, and it is an often-neglected element in discussion of preventative measures suitable for people who have already compromised their health (as in the first few paragraphs above) and who are candidates for this affliction.

Exercise, if performed regularly and if possessed of the three main components needed for optimum function (stretching, aerobics and relaxation) is a vital protective measure, as well as a tool to be used in recovery, once signs of returning energy are well established in the person with ME.

If you have ME severely and if physical exercise exhausts you further and causes pains and stiffness, then although you should for the time being avoid active exercising and anything too physical which might aggravate matters, there is no reason to avoid relaxation exercises or gentle stretching exercises (yoga type). There is much to be said for gentle stretching of tired and aching muscles as a means of reducing their acid waste load and retaining mobility.

What must be avoided in the active stages of ME are aerobic or physical 'toning'-type exercises.

Sleep

Sleep patterns can disrupt normal body cycles if they are disorganized and can enhance recovery if they come close to meeting the needs of the person. Current research at Charing Cross Hospital, as reported by Neville Hodgkinson in the *Sunday Times*, involves artificially induced sleep as a major part of the process of normalizing the health of people with ME. This will be a useful approach in some, although not the majority of cases.

In many cases I have found that, before ME struck, sleep played a relatively unimportant part in the routine, having been seen by a busy person, often stressed by deadlines and responsibilities, as a necessary nuisance. Is this one of the reasons why ME afflicts so large a proportion of the medical and nursing professions? 'Burn-out' is extremely common in these groups, and lack of adequate sleep accompanied by impossible workloads is another. The habit of taking a siesta, a nap after (or sometimes instead of) lunch, is to be encouraged in those facing 'burn-out', and it is vital for those who already have ME, as a part of their recovery programme.

Sleep disturbance is a major symptom of ME and needs to be dealt with as naturally as possible. Sleep should be restorative and in time, instead of waking feeling as tired as on lying down, the person with ME will begin to feel refreshed.

It is important that the normal cycles of sleep be encouraged and that dreaming be recalled. One of the clearest signs of vitamin B6 deficiency is lack of dream recall, and supplementing with this most useful of the B vitamins usually results in the remembering of dreams. Their significance or otherwise is not our present concern, but the very fact of remembering at least one of the night's dreams indicates that enough B6 is entering the system.

Standard drug-based sleeping tablets should be avoided if possible. Most such forms of medication are effective for no more than a few weeks and some are addictive. Even when effective the sleep produced has little relationship to a natural sleep pattern, with its cycles and phases such as REM (rapid eye movement) sleep. Unnatural (drug-induced) sleep is not as a rule refreshing sleep. While no one is yet quite sure why we need REM sleep so much, we do know that removing it from the sleep cycle, as drugs do, seriously reduces the value of such sleep.

Sleep experts Drs Philip Goldberg and Daniel Kaufman (in their book *Natural Sleep*, 1978) discuss the use of sleeping tablets after the first few weeks of use: 'The individual may, because he believes the drug is putting him to sleep, actually be able to relax enough so that he can doze off. But the pill itself isn't doing a thing. On the contrary, the pills are probably going to disturb the pattern of his sleep, and his sleep is probably going to be far more rotten because he's taking them.'

Dr Herbert Sheldon, quoted in the same book, states: 'Drugs do not produce sleep . . . In sleep the body is normally engaged in its most efficient reparative and building processes; in narcosis (drug-induced sleep) it is engaged in resisting and throwing off poison. . . . The first conserves energy, the second wastes energy. A night of sleep prepares us for normal function; narcosis leaves the digestive organs weak – there is nausea, a furred tongue, loss of appetite, dyspepsia, sometimes jaundice.' Hardly what the person with ME needs.

Coming off sleeping tablets can be a major problem, needing as it does months of weaning and often of detoxification. One recommended method is to withdraw one clinical dose of the sleeping tablet (the amount taken at night) once every week until natural sleep is once more enjoyed. Use of natural nutrients such as tryptophan (one of the amino acids from which protein is manufactured in the body) can effectively induce the drowsy state which leads so nicely to sleep.

Tryptophan is also a useful anti-depressant and relaxant, and can be used by anyone who finds going off to sleep difficult. It helps less in cases where going to sleep is easy but sleep is not lasting. A combination of tryptophan and other nutrients which enhance sleep (calcium, vitamin B6) is found in a product marketed through health food stores as Somnamin (Larkhall Laboratories) and this is suggested if an aid to sleeping is required. It is non-toxic, non-addictive and does not result in a drugged false sleep, and it does not interfere with REM (dream state) sleep. Tryptophan (and its co-factors) are taken half an hour before retiring.

Relaxation exercises as described in Chapter 10 are another method of inducing the preliminary drowsiness which is often lacking in the exhausted person with ME who just can't sleep. Learning to direct the mind towards the achievement of muscular and mental relaxation is sometimes all that is needed to start the process of sleep back towards normal.

A siesta should be taken after the midday meal, and this can be for anything from half-an-hour to three hours. I suggest that you go to bed and sleep at siesta time and not sit and watch TV or read. A deep refreshing midday sleep allows the rest of the day to be faced more effectively.

Other Environmental Factors

The phenomenon of 'sick building' syndrome is a twentieth-century health hazard which can make a home or an office a major element in the health, or lack of it, of its inhabitants. Over-insulation (and the materials used in insulation), accompanied by lack of free circulation of air – often resulting from sealed windows – can play a large part in feelings of fatigue.

Air-conditioning and heating systems can likewise add to the problem unless well designed (ducts correctly sited etc.) and maintained. Modern humans living in industrialized city environments spend upwards of 90 per cent of their lives indoors and so such influences are of some importance.

The mean temperature of a home or office is more likely to be efficient and comfortable if the temperature is around 68°F/20°C than if it is higher, which is customarily the case. Schoolchildren have been shown to function best at a temperature of 61°F/16°C.

The humidity (amount of water in the air) of living and working rooms is a key element in feelings of general exhaustion and lethargy if it rises above 55 per cent. The optimum level for feeling well and functioning efficiently is anywhere between 45 and 55 per cent humidity. Modern centrally heated rooms with double or triple glazing often fall to an amazing 3 per cent humidity (desert humidity is seldom below 20 per cent) and at this degree of dryness upper respiratory symptoms are frequent.

The movement of air in rooms in which we spend much time is another factor which needs consideration. Stagnant air results in feelings of heaviness, headaches and lethargy. If windows cannot be opened then regular excursions to fresh air are called for.

Residual pollution in the air of homes or offices reduces the levels of negative ions (which make us feel livelier) and increases positive ionization (which makes us feel sluggish). Positive ionization can contribute to the feeling of exhaustion attendant on living in modern buildings. It results from chemical gases released from synthetic materials used in construction and furnishings and from a host of household cleaning materials, from air pollution and stagnant air, smoke and smog, the operation of machines such as TV, and from air conditioning (positive ionization also results from impending storms and prevailing winds of course). The purchase of a negative air ionizer is suggested for every room in the home, since these are now inexpensive and compact (most weigh under a kilo).

The acquisition of full-spectrum light is also of importance to all of us, and this may mean sitting by an open window for periods of up to two hours each day if ill-health makes going outdoors difficult. Or it is possible to install lighting which carries with it the full spectrum of natural sunlight. Without this, a wide collection of symptoms, including 'nervous exhaustion' and general irritability, can result.

It is now well established that a number of viral, fungal or bacterial agents can be circulated via inefficient ventilation and heating systems if stagnant water or contamination of the air is a factor. A number of outbreaks of legionnaire's disease have been attributed to this cause. In the USA a modern Florida laboratory and office complex had to be redesigned after only two years of use when half of the 600 workers using it became ill (metallic tastes in their mouth, contact lenses changing colour, feelings of lethargy, headaches and skin rashes etc.). The cause was found to be circulating spores of animal-based fungi which were being sucked into the ventilation system from a veterinary unit in the complex. Homes can be equally dangerous and anyone who lives in one which has a tendency towards damp or mould, and who also has evidence of candida albicans overgrowth (see Chapter 6), should seriously consider moving house.

None of the environmental factors mentioned here are in themselves the cause of ME, yet all can contribute to the feelings of ill-health and exhaustion which it carries. Those with ME need to consider the home and workplace (assuming they are well enough to work) as possible factors in their illness and recovery programme, and deal with those elements which are capable of being addressed, including ventilation, humidity, air movement, temperature, ionization and full-spectrum light, as well as paying attention to the possible influence of mould, damp etc.

REFERENCES

The Beat Fatigue Workbook, Chaitow, L., Thorsons, Wellingborough 1988.
Natural Sleep, Goldberg, P., Kaufman, D., Rodale, Emmaus, Pa 1978.

Time Magazine, Health and Fitness section (on sick buildings), 6 June 1988.
' "Yuppie Flu" Is All in the Mind, Say Doctors', Hodgkinson, N., *Sunday Times*, 17 July 1988.

Part II

THE HEALING OF ME

---

9 Dietary and Supplementation Strategies

The dietary pattern which I will suggest in this chapter may require modification to take account of food sensitivities, intolerances and allergies. If any of the recommended foods are not acceptable for such reasons, or for reasons of personal taste, then obviously it is not intended that you ignore the messages from your body. Simply remove the foods from the menu.

The dietary recommendations will try to encompass the overall nutritional requirements of someone with ME. They are immune-system enhancing, have anti-candida (and sometimes antiviral) elements, and are useful for someone with hypoglycaemia. Within the framework of the suggested guidelines in this dietary pattern, however, there is much room for variation. It does not, in other words, need to be boring and irksome to eat correctly. You are allowed to enjoy your food as well as allowing it to do you good.

The common threads in a hypoglycaemic diet, an anti-candida diet and an immune-system enhancing diet, are that they all demand a very low sugar and low refined carbohydrate intake, a moderate fat intake, an adequate protein intake and a very high complex carbohydrate intake.

Candida as Part of the Problem

In addition, if candida is a part of the ME picture in your case (see Chapter 6) then it is assumed that your body will have become sensitized to yeast products. For this reason it is suggested that foods based on fermentation (wines, vinegar, miso etc.) or which are yeast-based (mushrooms, Marmite etc.) or which might be expected to contain high levels of mould, spores or fungi (cheese, dried fruit, tea etc.) should all be avoided for a period of several months, until the candida activity is well under control and an element of desensitization has taken place through lack of contact with these substances.

In the early stages (first 3–4 weeks) of following this diet I suggest that anyone with an obvious candida problem should not eat any fruit and more importantly, should not drink any fruit juice. This is because of the relatively high natural sugar content of fruits and the rapid absorption of these sugars when the fruit is juiced.

This restriction may be relaxed after the first month, with the gradual introduction of fruits, although melons should continue to be avoided until recovery is well under way.

If candida is not part of the problem then these specific recommendations relating to fermentation-based, or yeast-derived, foods and to fruit, do not apply.

A Word about Supplements

The supplements which are suggested for the person with ME are designed to perform several tasks. Most are specifically immune-system enhancers, whereas others have different roles to play (aiding digestion, speeding detoxification, enhancing protein supply etc.). Some have anti-candida and antiviral potentials and some enhance the way the body metabolizes and deals with sugars (chromium for example).

There are a lot of supplements to be taken. This may require some getting used to, and I suggest that you look on supplements not as medicines but as the concentrated foods which they are.

In cases where candida is operating it is necessary to avoid yeast-based supplements, and this is possible by purchasing specific brands of nutrients which guarantee that they are not extracted from or derived from fermentation or yeast.

Some nutrients, such as the amino acids (from which protein is made) and enzymes, need to be taken away from meal times, on their own with water. Other nutrients should be taken at meal times (during or after) unless specific instructions to the contrary are given. In some instances divided doses are better than just one large dose. Such advice is given in the text with the dosage suggestions.

Do Diet and Supplementation Really Help?

Without doubt they do. A most dramatic personal illustration of the value of this approach was that of Mr E.M., a young civil servant who consulted me in 1982, before I was aware of ME. His symptoms of almost total exhaustion accompanied by a host of classic ME symptoms, ranging from blurred vision to digestive distress and light-headedness, had started seven years earlier after he developed gastroenteritis whilst on holiday (treated with broad-spectrum antibiotics). His condition was so severe that he could function for only brief periods before collapsing again with total exhaustion. He had been through the medical mill including being hospitalized twice, as well as having tried rotation diets to reduce food sensitivity symptoms.

At that time I treated him for what I assumed to be

candida overgrowth, with a dietary programme, antifungal nutrients (described below) and general supplementation to support immune function (vitamins A, B1, B2,
B3, B5, B6, calcium, magnesium, manganese and vitamin
C).

Improvement began almost immediately and symptoms
were relieved by about 50 per cent after six months (this was
now seven and a half years since their onset). Relapses
occurred whenever he strayed from the dietary pattern and
introduced yeast-based foods (see below) or anything too
sugary. This proved to him in the most direct manner just
how much the diet and supplements meant to his recovery,
and induced a steadily increasing compliance to the programme. Eighteen months after beginning his dietary
programme he was so much better overall that he felt no
further need to see me, and was able to adhere much less
strictly to the diet.

The case of Sue Finlay, which is briefly described in
Chapter 6, is another example of the enormous value of the
use of the diet and supplement programme in supporting
immune function, retarding candida activity and allowing
ME to start healing.

Basic Guidelines – Foods to Avoid

*The person with ME, with or without candida, with or without
hypoglycaemia, should avoid the following:*

- All sugar, whether white, brown or shades between.
  This includes honey.
- Sweets, glacé fruits, jellies, jams, pickles, sauces,
  preserved fruits and anything else which has 'hidden'
  sugars.
- All alcohol of any sort.
- Anything made from refined (white) flour products
  (buns, cakes, pastries, crackers, biscuits, pasta etc.).

These can be safely and beneficially replaced with foods made from wholegrain cereals (brown pasta, wholegrain bread, etc.).

- Any foods or drinks containing colouring, flavouring or preservatives.
- Frozen vegetables which contain sugar (peas and many others).
- Breakfast cereals containing sugars or made with refined flours.
- Fruit juice (unless diluted 50/50 with water and sipped slowly).
- Stimulants which trigger the release of sugar in the body such as tea, coffee, cola, cigarettes and alcohol.
- Any meat or fish dishes which have been cured, smoked, preserved, pickled or in any way processed. This includes sausages, salami, bacon.

The person with candida should also avoid:
Fruit (for the first month or so); milk (because of its high milk sugar content); all yeast-derived or fermented foods. The latter include: bread (apart from non-yeasted varieties), mushrooms, soya sauce, Indian or China tea, nuts and seeds (unless fresh and free of rancidity and mould), cider, beer, ginger ale, wine etc., cheese (apart from cottage cheese), all malted products, vinegar of any sort, sauerkraut, pickles, relishes and sauces, anything containing monosodium glutamate (widely found in Chinese restaurant foods), anything cooked in breadcrumbs, anything containing citric acid (usually yeast derived), and for the same reason most canned or frozen citrus drinks, and mayonnaise. You should only choose multi-vitamin/multi-mineral/B-complex vitamins/individual B vitamins/selenium supplements that are *guaranteed from a yeast-free source*.

Antibiotics should be avoided by anyone with candida unless absolutely unavoidable. Meats and poultry which might be from sources in which antibiotics are used should also be avoided.

The person with hypoglycaemia should avoid:
The foods listed as undesirable for the person with ME, as well as fruit. They should try to eat little and often, with a last meal at bedtime and a pre-breakfast snack waiting at the bedside (seeds such as sunflower or pumpkin, or almonds, or natural live yogurt).

General Recommendations and Diet for the Person with ME

1 All fruits and vegetables should be organically grown if at all possible.
2 Tinned, commercially frozen and pre-packaged foods should in general be avoided.
3 Avoid artificial sweeteners (aspartame etc.).
4 Irradiated and microwave cooked foods should be avoided as enzyme and other nutrient levels are severely compromised by these methods.
5 Foods to which have been added colouring, preservatives, flavouring or other chemical agents should be avoided.
6 Smoked foods should be avoided.
7 Try to replace red (muscle) meat with fish, poultry (without skin), or game (rabbit, venison etc.), or organ meat (spleen, liver, kidney etc.), or with vegetarian protein combinations in which a grain (e.g. brown rice, wholemeal pasta) and a pulse (e.g. lentils, chickpeas, beans) are combined in a dish or at the same meal to provide a complete range of amino acids.
8 Of the dairy produce available avoid most, except for live natural yogurt and low-fat and cottage cheese.

9 Use only mono-unsaturated oils in cooking (first pressing olive oil or sesame oil are best) and on salads. Avoid direct heating of oils if possible.

10 Approximately 2 to 3 pints of liquid should be consumed daily and this should be spring water (avoid tap water unless filtered) or juice derived from the cooking of vegetables. Avoid carbonated drinks or those which have flavouring or sweetening added.

11 Use only small amounts of salt for cooking and flavouring, relying more on herbs such as garlic, thyme, rosemary etc.

12 Avoid roasting or frying foods and try to eat meals when the food is neither very hot nor very cold.

Menu Examples

Breakfast. Choose one or two of the following:

1 Raw breakfast cereal mixture (muesli). Any sugar-free wholegrain cereal foods including brown rice, millet, wheat, rye, barley, oats (including oatmeal and oat bran) or buckwheat may be used in a homemade muesli which can be soaked or dry and raw. Whole or cracked or flaked cereals are mixed with seeds and (after the first few weeks) fruit. Seeds which are suitable for addition to such dishes include pumpkin, sesame, sunflower, linseed etc. Wheatgerm and/or freshly milled nuts (almonds and walnuts are best) may be added as well. Muesli-type mixtures may be moistened with sugar-free soya milk or natural yogurt.

2 Cooked breakfast cereal mixture. This may be made by combining at least five of the following: barley, wheat, millet, linseed, buckwheat, brown rice, oats, sunflower seeds, pumpkin seeds, sesame seeds which

have been ground in a food processor. Add 2 to 3 cups of this mixture to one pint (2½ cups) of cold water together with a teaspoonful of salt substitute (potassium chloride from health food stores). Cook this on medium heat until it thickens, stirring frequently (5 minutes or so), and serve warm with added yogurt and (after the first few weeks, fruit). Season with cinnamon if desired or ground cashew nuts.

3 Variations can be introduced in which two or three of the above cereals such as millet and buckwheat and a seed such as linseed are either combined whole and soaked overnight in a little water to soften them, or ground together in a processor or nut mill and eaten with soya milk or natural yogurt.

4 Oatmeal or millet flake porridge with cinnamon or grated nuts, using no honey and no sugar.

5 Three times a week have two eggs any style except fried or raw (raw eggs contain a chemical which destroys biotin, the B vitamin vital for control of candida).

6 Yeast- and sugar-free wholegrain toast or rice or oat cakes with butter and sugarless jam.

7 Oat or rice pancakes (sugar free), and sugarless jam.

8 Kedgeree (brown rice and fish dish) or any other fish dish (not smoked, cured or fried).

9 Natural live yogurt flavoured with freshly milled nuts or cinnamon.

10 When fruit is again available (after a month on the programme) introduce those with high enzyme content such as papaya, mango, pineapple, avocado, kiwi fruit etc. as well as basic apples, pears, peaches, plums, grapes etc. Dried fruit is high in mould content and is seldom anything other than chemically dried. It should be avoided.

To drink, herbal teas – at least some of these – are acceptable if freshly picked and dried. Some are high in caffeine and tannin and should be avoided. The best are Japanese green tea, Rooibos (redbush) tea from southern Africa, and camomile tea. Coffee substitutes may be used if these are free from sugar and (at least for the ME patient with candida problems) if they have no yeast-derived elements.

Between-meal snacks. Seeds (sunflower, pumpkin etc.) and fresh, unsalted, unroasted, nuts (walnuts, almonds, pecans) are ideal snacks for anyone with hypoglycaemia who has to eat little and often. Others should not need such snacks.

Main meal (1). One main meal should be a high-protein meal including fish, poultry (no skin), game or organ meat in any form except roasted or fried, or a vegetarian pulse/grain combination for complete protein (cooked rice or wheat and lentils or chickpeas or other beans in a soup, 'nutroast' or other combination).

These foods should be eaten with a selection of freshly (lightly) cooked vegetables and/or salad vegetables. If digestion is a problem then the lightly cooked vegetable selection is more acceptable than salad at first, and methods of cooking should ensure retention of nutrients.

One of the best ways of achieving this is by stir (wok) frying (using small amounts of olive or sesame oil), in which high heat and minimum time are involved (together with constant agitation of the food) in order to tenderize the vegetables without losing food value. Steaming and lightly boiling are also acceptable methods of tenderizing vegetables.

Dress vegetables with olive oil and lemon juice on serving to add flavour and reduce oxidation. Flavour with salt substitute or herbs including garlic.

Sea vegetables (seaweed) are now available dried in speciality and health stores and these are nutritious and tasty. Cooked rice, wholemeal pasta or pulses are suitable additional foods to add to such meals.

109

If candida is not a problem then fermented soya curd (soya cheese or tofu) is an excellent source of high-quality protein which is easily digested and capable of being prepared in a variety of ways.

Main meal (2). The other main meal should include some protein, or a complex carbohydrate mixture, and a raw salad (if digestion is up to coping with this).

Salads should include a selection of raw vegetables currently in season such as cabbage, cauliflower, artichoke, tomato, sprouted seeds (alfalfa, mung bean, fenugreek etc.), fennel, celery, kale, chives, chicory, radish, mustard and cress, purslaine, watercress, peppers, onions, parsley, mint, endive, lettuce, spinach, beetroot (grated raw, or cooked, but without vinegar), turnip (grated), spring onions, spring or clove garlic, mushrooms (not candida patients) etc., etc.

Choose four or five of the above, selecting for availability, freshness, colour combinations (eye-appeal is important) and flavour. Dress lightly with olive oil and lemon juice.

The salad can be eaten with a protein dish (meat, fish or vegetarian pulse/rice mixture or with cottage cheese or nuts and seeds). A jacket potato can be eaten with this meal if no meat or fish or cheese is included (they combine poorly).

All food should be thoroughly chewed and eaten slowly. If appetite is poor then soups can be used initially, but in the long run the lighter the cooking the more of the vital nutrients and enzymes will be retained.

Drink only a little water or herbal teas with meals.

Try to avoid combinations in which a concentrated protein (fish, meat etc.) is eaten at the same meal as a concentrated carbohydrate (potato, bread) or fat-rich foods. Careful food combining helps the digestive process.

A week's menu. This might look something like the following (suggestion only):

Breakfast	4 mornings – muesli or cooked cereal dish and yogurt. Herb tea.
	3 mornings – boiled eggs and rice or oat cakes. Herb tea.
Lunch	3 days – fish dish (grilled or steamed) and lightly cooked vegetables.
	2 days – poultry (once as a soup and once with lightly cooked vegetables and side salad).
	1 day – vegetarian pulse/cereal combination and vegetables or pasta dish (wholemeal pasta) with cheese.
	1 day – game or organ meat (rabbit, venison or liver) and vegetables and side salad.
Evening	3 days – mixed salad and cottage cheese, chicken, omelette or fish.
	2 days – vegetarian pulse/rice/tofu (bean curd) dish with salad and steamed or stir-fried vegetables and Japanese seaweed.
	2 days – small salad and egg, followed by soup (vegetable and brown pasta or bean or chicken) or lunch-style meal.

If candida is not a problem then the selection of cheeses can widen and fruit can play a larger part in the diet. This could allow for more interesting meals with fruit desserts as well as different cheeses with salads. Cooked cheese should always be avoided for digestive reasons.

Pulses require special attention in their cooking. The ideal is to soak before cooking and to discard the water used for this. For those with sensitive digestions pulses should be partly cooked and then have the water changed before completing the cooking. This eliminates enzymes which produce flatulence for some people, thus making the eating of pulses unpleasant instead of the delicious/nutritious experience it ought to be. The kidney bean family should always be soaked for at least five hours, and then boiled hard in fresh water before being reduced to a simmer.

As a general rule if a cooked protein dish is eaten at one meal then a salad should be eaten at the other, unless an effort is made to adopt the American pattern of having a salad of some sort at each meal.

If hypoglycaemia is part of the problem then the between-meal snacks are important additional sources of nutrients and a late-night snack of yogurt or an egg is suggested.

There is an endless selection of acceptable foods and the acquisition of recipe books which encourage low-fat, low-salt, wholefood cooking (with some vegetarian dishes as well) can swiftly perk up tired and jaded palates.

Antiviral (Herpes-Type Viruses) Nutrition

Some of the major viral suspects in the causation of ME include members of the herpes virus family, including cytomegalovirus, varicella-zoster virus and Epstein-Barr virus.

Herpes viruses have nearly identical appearances when viewed under an electron microscope and share many similar characteristics. They all contain DNA and their components are synthesized inside the nucleus of infected cells. In most cases long-term immunity from further infection is not achieved after the initial infection because of one of the most important characteristics of herpes viruses, their ability to become latent after infection. They can take refuge in the body and become reactivated at times of lowered immune function, when conditions are ideal for them. Since one or other of the herpes virus family may be active in people with ME, and since it is known that some of the herpes viruses can be modified in their activity, and prevented from reactivation, by dietary means, some specific foods are recommended and others viewed as undesirable in anything but small amounts.

This nutritional strategy, to which I alluded briefly in Chapter 7, was discovered accidentally in the research laboratories of the University of California, Los Angeles, where Dr Christopher Kagan first noticed that when herpes simplex viruses were being grown in culture dishes this process could be speeded up if the amino acid arginine was added. This amino acid is very similar to another of these protein fractions, the essential amino acid lysine. If lysine is given to herpes viruses in a culture dish their growth is not speeded but rather is slowed or stopped.

Kagan wondered whether this strategy might not also work in humans, and in 1974 he conducted the first study of this approach on 45 patients. It was found that doses of around 1000 milligrams of lysine daily suppressed recurrence of herpes outbreaks. It is thought that the virus may mistake lysine for arginine, and that this stops or slows their replication.

In practice this has been found to be a very effective strategy for people with herpes simplex infection, who can alter their dietary intake to favour lysine-rich foods, at the same time as reducing the intake of arginine-rich foods. The alternative is to take supplemental lysine.

The only unfortunate element of the dietary approach is that most of the foods which are rich in arginine (and therefore relatively undesirable for people with herpes virus) are among those most desirable from a general health viewpoint. Nuts in particular (some varieties) are very rich in arginine and poor in lysine content.

A strategy which tries to include lysine-rich food and which moderates arginine-rich food, at the same time as supplementing modest amounts of lysine, is the one I

113

recommend. The choice of foods should be such that those arginine-rich foods which are desirable for general nutrition are included but not as a major part of the diet.

This approach will only be of value to the person with ME if there is persistent or recurrent viral activity. Evidence for this might come from periodic reactivation of slight fever, flu-like symptoms, sore throats and swollen glands etc. as well as the usual ME symptoms.

Lysine-Rich and Arginine-Rich Foods

The following foods are *rich in lysine* and therefore helpful in reducing herpes virus activity. (They are listed in order of richness of lysine. The figure in each case indicates the average excess of lysine over arginine and therefore the relative beneficial amount of that substance available to you):

Fresh fish	950 milligrams in 4 ounce serving
Tinned fish	880 milligrams in 4 ounce serving
Chicken	740 milligrams in 4 ounce serving
Beef	720 milligrams in 4 ounce serving
Goat's milk	520 milligrams in 1 cup
Cow's milk	420 milligrams in 1 cup
Lamb	420 milligrams in 4 ounce serving
Cooked mung beans	410 milligrams in ½ cup
Pork	380 milligrams in 4 ounce serving
All types of cheese	280 milligrams in 1 ounce serving

Cooked beans   250 milligrams in ½ cup
Cottage cheese   220 milligrams in ½ cup
Sprouted mung beans   210 milligrams in ½ cup
Brewer's yeast   190 milligrams in 1 table-
                                 spoonful
Shell fish   170 milligrams in 4 ounce
                                 serving
Soya products   130 milligrams in ½ cup
Eggs   120 milligrams in 1 egg

Those foods *rich in arginine* and therefore *not desirable* in any
quantity for anyone with persistent or latent herpes virus
infection include (in order of excess of arginine over lysine):

Hazelnuts   2250 milligrams in ½ cup
Brazil nuts   2110 milligrams in ½ cup
Peanuts   2060 milligrams in ½ cup
Walnuts   810 milligrams in ½ cup
Almonds   710 milligrams in ½ cup
Cocoa and chocolate   650 milligrams in ½ cup
Peanut butter   510 milligrams in 2 tablespoons
Sesame seeds   450 milligrams in ½ cup
Cashew nuts   420 milligrams in ½ cup
Carob powder   310 milligrams in ½ cup
Coconut   290 milligrams in ½ cup
Pistachio nuts   240 milligrams in ½ cup
Buckwheat flour   230 milligrams in ½ cup
Chickpeas   210 milligrams in ½ cup
Brown rice   200 milligrams in ½ cup
Pecan nuts   180 milligrams in ½ cup
Wholewheat bread   160 milligrams in 4 slices
Oatmeal (cooked)   130 milligrams in ½ cup
Raisins   130 milligrams in ½ cup
Sunflower seeds   120 milligrams in ½ cup

115

An eating strategy based on these figures requires some thought because quite obviously not all the foods listed are as richly endowed with the dominant nutrient (lysine or arginine) as others. There should not necessarily therefore be a total abandonment of any foods in which arginine dominates, simply a modification of intake.

If you were to eat a 4 ounce portion of fish this would have some 950 milligrams of lysine in excess of arginine. If at the same meal you were to eat half a cup of brown rice, which contains around 200 milligrams of arginine in excess of lysine, the net benefit (lysine over arginine) would still be 700 milligrams. This would be highly desirable from the point of view of controlling herpes virus activity despite eating the relatively arginine-rich rice.

If, however, you rounded out the meal with half a cupful of hazelnuts which contains a massive 2250 milligrams of arginine in excess of lysine, the deficit in terms of too much arginine at the end of this meal would be 1550 milligrams of arginine. This would be very undesirable and could encourage herpes reactivation.

We can see from the lists that rice contains slightly more arginine than lysine, and beans more lysine than arginine. If in a combination dish both beans (high lysine) and rice (high arginine) are eaten, a relatively neutral result is achieved with neither dominating. This is important since we need whole grains, and it is by careful choice of the balancing foods that we can continue to enjoy these without creating an environment in which herpes will decide to flourish again.

It is considered by researchers that we need some 1500 milligrams of additional lysine over arginine intake daily, in order to hold herpes viruses in check. If a rough calculation of the foods you eat seems to indicate too much arginine then supplementation can make up the difference. Lysine is available in 500 milligram tablets from health food stores and this should be supplemented to ensure that there is a constant excess of lysine.

One of the factors which protects lysine levels in the body is vitamin C (together with associated nutrients with which it is found in nature called bioflavonoids). When lysine is supplemented vitamin C should also be taken. This has a further benefit in allowing excess lysine to be converted into another amino acid, carnitine, which is discussed below in relation to its usefulness in enhancing energy production.

By reasonable care over food selections (easy on the hazel and brazil nuts, no chocolate and plenty of fish and beans etc.) as well as moderate lysine supplementation this strategy of inhibiting herpes virus activity need not be arduous.

Supplementation of 1500 milligrams of L-lysine is suggested daily for anyone with evidence of continuing herpes virus activity, together with some care over food selection. In conjunction, the same amount of vitamin C (ideally this should be a form which states 'with bio-flavonoids') should be taken. *This amino acid supplement should (as with all amino acids) be taken away from meal times in divided doses with water.*

The various nutritional guidelines given above should be modified to your needs. If allergy or sensitivity exists to any of the foods mentioned then it is of the greatest importance that you avoid such foods, at least for the time being. I have not described the complexities of elimination and rotation diets which are used by clinical ecologists and nutritional allergy specialists to identify such foods. Allergies and their treatment are beyond the scope of this book, but anyone with ME should be aware of a possible connection and should consult an appropriate adviser for guidance and treatment.

If candida is a part of the problem then the specialized alterations to the diet which this calls for should be instituted. The same applies to the possibility of hypo-glycaemia. You have also just seen that dietary changes may be called for in response to virus activity.

Enough Protein?

If candida overgrowth, viral activity, hypoglycaemia and/or allergic reactions are concurrently in evidence, then the pattern of eating could be very restricted indeed. If any combination of these is a factor in ME then it is of the greatest importance that adequate protein be consumed. This may present a problem for anyone with a compro-mised digestive system and I therefore recommend the use of what are called 'free-form' amino acids in supplemental form.

We all need to find in our food each day a selection of essential amino acids from which we can make all the other amino acids and from this raw material restore and build the tissues and cells of the body. There are eight (some say ten) essential amino acids which have to be present in our food and which, in order to be of any use to us, need to be adequately digested. Unless these are separated from each other (they arrive in food in chains) so that they are 'free' we cannot use them to construct new tissues.

Because many people with ME have inadequate digestive function it is useful to take ready-prepared amino acids, which the body can then alter to make up the complete set of twenty or so amino acids which form part of everything in the body.

Between 5 and 15 grams daily of free-form amino acids (the whole complex ideally or just the essential ones) should be taken half-an-hour before or an hour-and-a-half after meals with water. I have given addresses of manufacturers and distributors of these and other nutritional supplements in the Resources section.

If lysine (or any other amino acid such as tryptophan, to aid sleep) is being supplemented then this should be taken at a separate time from the free-form amino acid complex. This is to ensure adequate absorption and to avoid competition for uptake by the bloodstream.

Supplements for ME

In order to enhance immune function the following nutrients should be supplemented for at least six months and ideally until adequate energy levels are well established and health is good. If candida is part of the picture then yeast-free sources need to be ensured. Some guidance on this is given in the text.

Antioxidants

1   A combination of vitamins A (in the form of beta carotene), C, E and the mineral selenium provide a good basic formulation of antioxidants which enhance immune function. Nature's Best (see Resources section) produce a *Beta Carotene, C, E and Selenium* tablet with a good dosage balance. One or two of these should be taken daily with food.

2   It is now known that the major enzyme antioxidants can be supplemented orally to good effect and I suggest that between 4 and 6 capsules of *OxyPlex* *(contains glutathione peroxidase, methionine reductase, catalase and superoxide dismutase)* be taken every day on an empty stomach. These are marketed by BioCare and their address is in the Resources section.

Immune-system enhancers

1   The B-vitamins are essential for sound immune functioning. Not only should several of these be taken individually (see below) but the entire complex should be supplemented in a formulation with high potency. Nature's Best supply a *B-100 Complex* tablet and one of these daily is suggested with food. For those with candida a yeast-free B-complex is available from Bio-Health (address in Resources section) and 2 of these daily with meals is suggested.

2   Additional intake of *vitamin B6 (pyridoxine)* is desirable and this should be taken (50 to 100 milligrams daily) at a separate time from the B-complex supplement.

3   *Zinc* is essential for the healthy function of the thymus gland, a major component of the immune system. A daily intake of 20 to 40 milligrams is needed. If zinc orotate in doses of 100 milligrams (Larkhall Laboratories) is used this provides the body with about 15 to 20 grams of zinc. This should be taken with meals. If zinc picolinate is available this is known to be one of the best absorbed forms.

4   The minerals *calcium* and *magnesium* are useful additions to an immune-system enhancing programme. These are taken in doses of 1000 and 500 milligrams respectively, ideally at bedtime.

5   *Essential fatty acids* in the form of oil of evening primrose help to enhance immune function and 1000 to 1500 milligrams daily of this should be taken with food, in divided doses.

6   If there is ongoing viral activity, and during periods in which symptoms are worse, additional nutrients are required including: (a) *Vitamin C* in doses of up to 10 grams daily in divided doses. Higher doses are recommended if supervision from a health care professional is available, since it is now known that

introduction of vitamin C to bowel tolerance (in other words until diarrhoea starts) has the effect of 'saturating' the tissues with ascorbic acid (vitamin C) which has an antiviral and antibiotic action. (b) *Beta-carotene* (which the body turns into vitamin A) in doses of up to 200,000 iu daily. This form of vitamin A is completely non-toxic.

7 *A good formulation multi-mineral supplement* to ensure that balanced nutrition is maintained during this high supplementation period. These are available from health food stores.

8 *Lactobacillus acidophilus* as a means of repopulating the digestive tract with friendly bacteria which have antiviral and antibiotic properties as well as being themselves a source of B vitamins. Dosage is discussed below under the candida supplementation heading.

Other Digestive Aids

If digestion is poor the addition of enzymes to aid in digestion of the various foods eaten can be a major help. For assistance in protein digestion take proteolytic (protein-digesting) enzymes such as *bromelaine and papain* (sources in Resources section).

If dyspepsia is regularly felt after eating there may be a shortage of hydrochloric acid and this too can be supplemented. Nature's Best supply *betaine hydrochloride* and *pepsin* in tablet form for use at the beginning of meals.

Anti-Candida Supplementation

Supplementation in addition to the nutrients mentioned above is required if candida is a current problem for the person with ME. The specific additional nutrients include:

1 *High potency acidophilus* powder – a vital part of the

anti-candida programme. The brand recommended is
Superdophilus (G&G Supplies, see Resources section)
together with other lactobacilli such as *bifido factor* and
lactobacillus bulgaricus. Dosage for someone *with* candida
is a quarter teaspoonful of acidophilus powder in water
2 or 3 times daily away from mealtimes, and a quarter
teaspoonful each of bifido factor and bulgaricus in water
at a separate time from the acidophilus.

Additional aid to the digestive tract can be derived by
using symbiotic bacterial concentrates containing a
variety of cultures including streptococcus
thermophilus. These are available in a form called
ProBion from ISSS (see Resources).

2 500 microgrammes of *biotin*, a B vitamin, with food.
3 High potency *garlic* capsules (unless a great deal of raw
   garlic is being eaten) for its antifungal activity. Take 3 to
   6 capsules daily with meals. (KWAI brand
   recommended, from health stores.)
4 *Oleic acid*, which is simply the active portion of olive oil,
   is also antifungal. A dessertspoonful of oil daily on salad
   will provide this.
5 A non-nutrient extract of coconuts is caprylic acid which
   is a powerful antifungal agent and completely non-toxic
   (as it is not absorbed but simply passes through the gut
   killing yeast). The form recommended is *caprycin*
   (source BioCare, see Resources). Three time-release
   capsules should be taken with each meal. This product
   has the additional bonus of supplying calcium and
   magnesium to the body while it is killing off the yeast.
6 *Germanium* is discussed further in the section below
   dealing with energy enhancement. It has powerful
   antifungal properties and its supplementation is
   recommended at a dosage of not less than 100
   milligrams daily. It is expensive, however, and will
   continue to be so until a cheaper method of production

is developed. Sources are given in the Resources section.

7   *Aloe vera juice* is derived from the desert plant and it is an antifungal substance. Several teaspoonsful in water should be consumed daily (G&G Supplies).

The substances and nutrients in the above list should be used for not less than six months by anyone with a candida problem. I have found in many cases that this approach is often enough to make a considerable difference to anyone with ME. The return of energy and of a general feeling of being able to function again allows for a major step back towards normality.

Note. During periods of rapid yeast destruction the body is called on to detoxify the breakdown products of this process and this can lead to your feeling particularly seedy, nauseous and off-colour. The reaction is known as yeast 'die-off' or 'burn-off' and can last for some days or even weeks. The use of bifido factor (see above) and the general dietary strategies discussed earlier in the chapter should minimize this. Do not, however, stop the anti-candida programme as this is a critical stage of the treatment; if stopped suddenly it can lead to a rebound of the candida and even greater feelings of ill-health.

Energy Enhancing Nutrients

ME is nothing if it is not characterized by exhaustion, tiredness, fatigue. The answer to this is not to stimulate energy artificially but, as I have said in earlier chapters, to remove the obstacles to normal energy production and bodily function.

I have already briefly discussed the use of free-form amino acids and this is urged as part of an attempt to provide the raw materials from which energy is derived.

1   A dose of 5 to 15 grams daily of *free-form amino acids* in
    a balanced formulation which contains all the essential
    amino acids and those with which they are associated,
    in the correct ratios for immediate use by the body.
    Manufacturers and suppliers such as Nature's Best,
    Larkhall Laboratories, Nature's Flow and G&G
    Supplies are all recommended.

2   The amino acid *L-glutamine* is capable of passing
    through the blood-brain barrier where it is turned into
    glutamic acid, a detoxifier of ammonia in the brain
    and a supplier of energy to this most vital structure.
    Glutamic acid has been described by the great
    researcher into nutrition, Professor Roger Williams, as
    'the unique brain fuel'. A dosage of 200 to 300
    milligrams taken three times daily with water away
    from food is suggested, especially if concentration and
    memory are poor. A bonus from this supplementation
    is that glutamine reduces the desire for sugary foods
    and alcohol.

3   *Germanium*, which is suggested as an anti-candida
    nutrient, is also suggested for its remarkable energy-
    enhancing and cell oxygenation features. The dosage
    used for candida should not be less than 100
    milligrams daily, indefinitely. If ME is severe and
    energy very low then higher intake of organic
    germanium is desirable, up to 300 milligrams daily
    with food. This is, however, an expensive nutrient.

4   A major part in the energy-making cycle is played by
    a recently researched substance called *coenzyme Q10*,
    and this has been found to act beneficially on energy
    production when taken for some months. Its role is in
    the electron transport chain – a biochemical pathway
    in cellular respiration from which metabolic energy is
    derived. Little benefit is felt before six weeks of

supplementation at dosage levels of between 50 and 100 milligrams daily, with food.

5   Those people taking lysine to counteract viral activity will have an additional bonus because from this amino acid the body manufactures another amino acid called *carnitine*. Carnitine has remarkable functions in relation to the fat metabolism of the body in general, and more specifically in transferring fatty acids across the membranes of the cells of the body so that they can be used for energy production. Carnitine should be supplemented to enhance energy production if lysine is not being supplemented. Carnitine dosage should be at levels of 1 to 3 grams daily away from meals and taken with vitamin B6.

Nutrients for the Hypoglycaemic Condition

Glucose tolerance factor chromium should be supplemented along with the general anti-sugar/high complex carbo-hydrate/frequent meal strategy. A dose of between 500 microgrammes and 1 milligram is suggested daily. BioCare produce an *organic chromium complex* in liquid form which is highly recommended. Each drop contains 150 microgram-mes of chromium and so 3 to 4 drops daily are suggested.

Oral Chelation

If it is established that toxicity is a factor (see Chapter 5), it is necessary to employ appropriate tactics to help the body rid itself of heavy metal accumulations. Chelation is derived from the Greek word for a claw, and chelating agents – of which oatmeal porridge, pectin in apples and algin from seaweed are examples – act by grabbing or latching on to offending substances and eliminating them from the bowel.

The following combination – all available from any health food store – creates a formula which will do this efficiently on a self-help basis. Quantities given are for daily use, but you may prefer to mix a larger batch and keep it in the fridge.

4 grams lecithin
12 grams coarsely chopped sunflower seeds (a source of linoleic acid and potassium)
5 grams debittered brewer's yeast (a source of selenium, chromium and B vitamins). *NB* This should *not* be included if candida is part of the problem
2 grams bonemeal (a source of calcium and magnesium)
5 grams raw wheatgerm (a source of vitamin E)
500 milligrams vitamin C
100 iu vitamin E
25 grams zinc

Place these together in a blender and grind to a powder. Refrigerate and use in or with food.

In addition, an amino acid supplement – 1–1.5 grams daily of either methionine or cysteine – may be taken.

Intravenous chelation is not a self-help measure but requires expert professional attention – for address see Resources section.

General Support from Adaptogens

A class of substances which produce a non-specific supportive or defensive effect on the body, allowing it to withstand greater stress or toxicity than otherwise, have been termed adaptogens. These have been extensively researched, especially in Russia in relation to the space programme, where they are used to offer protection against radiation damage. They have a role to play for anyone who is severely ill or run down, where immune function is less than adequate.

The major adaptogens include *eleutherococcus senticosus* (Siberian ginseng), which is considered especially effective where prolonged physical or mental stress is involved. It is known to increase mental alertness and to have immune-potentiating qualities. It is milder in action than panax ginseng (the Korean version) which can be overstimulating. Recommended dosage for general adaptogen support is 2 to 4 grams of dried root three times daily or 2 to 4 millilitres of fluid extract three times daily.

Other adaptogens include royal jelly and pollen extracts which can be used for general purposes if desired.

Raw Glandular Concentrates

Support of the endocrine (hormonal/glandular) systems of the body can be derived from use of raw glandular concentrates derived from beef or sheep organs. Use of thymus extract has been shown to prevent this vital gland from becoming defective during chronic ill-health. Supplementation with thymus, adrenal and spleen concentrates is a useful method of supporting these organs with vital nutrients and hormones which these concentrates retain and which are capable of absorption from the digestive system intact. Suppliers are listed in the Resources section and dosages are usually in the region of 300 to 900 milligrams daily of each. These are not suitable for vegetarians or anyone allergic to beef or sheep meat.

This nutritional programme is the basis of recovery from ME. It requires effort and dedication and a great deal of patience. Combined with the stress-reducing/relaxation/visualization methods described in the next chapter, it has brought many people with ME back to relative normality over a period of months or years.

REFERENCES

Amino Acids in Therapy, Chaitow, L., Thorsons, Wellingborough 1986.

The Amino Revolution, Erdmann, R., Jones, M., Century, London 1987.

A World without AIDS, Chaitow, L., Martin, S., Thorsons, Wellingborough 1988.

Candida Albicans: Could Yeast Be Your Problem? Chaitow, L., Thorsons, Wellingborough 1986.

Internal Medicine, editor-in-chief Stein, J. H., Little Brown, Boston 1983.

Maximum Immunity, Weiner, M., Gateway Books, Bath 1987.

Nutritional Influences on Illness, Werbach, M., Third Line Press, Tarzana, California 1987.

Nutritional Medicine, Davies, S., Stewart, A., Pan Books, London 1987.

'Oxygen Nutrition for Super Health (Germanium)', Levine, S., *Journal of Orthomolecular Nutrition*, vol. 1, no. 3, pp. 145–8, 1986.

Stop Your Herpes Now, Healthworks Medical Group, South Laguna, California 1981.

Textbook of Natural Medicine, Pizzorno, J., Murray, M., JBCNM, Seattle 1987.

Win Against Herpes and AIDS, Snead, E. L., Metro Medical Publications, San Antonio, Texas 1987.

10 Harnessing Mind-Power

There is for many people a direct connection between stress (as they perceive it) and:

- A build-up of muscular tension.
- Altered breathing patterns (sometimes including hyperventilation).
- Changes in blood chemistry resulting from this.
- Reduced energy levels associated with tension in the muscles.
- Increased levels of anxiety as a result of all of the above.
- Greater degrees of 'arousal' (we become more easily upset).
- Even poorer stress-coping ability and lowered immune function (evidenced by increased susceptibility to viral and other infection).
- Greater likelihood of allergies (and therefore even more immune suppression).
- Added to this, all the other consequences of virus infection, candida infection, and resultant nutritional deficits and toxicities, as well as digestive complications.

This connection between 'stress' and ill-health can be altered at a number of points along the way:

1 We can learn to cope better in response to stress.
2 We can learn to relax tight tense muscles, and to stretch these gently and safely, thus saving energy (it uses a great deal of energy just keeping a muscle tense).
3 We can learn breathing methods which reduce the chance of the nasty consequences of hyperventilation.
4 We can learn to apply the healing potential of the mind through techniques such as relaxation, guided imagery or visualization (also known as therapeutic meditation).

By doing these things we can effectively allow the self-healing, homoeostatic mechanisms of the body to operate freely, protecting against a decline into ill-health, raising immune function levels, and regaining health if this is already impaired. (Such a desirable result will be achieved more positively if we are at the same time supplying the body with those nutrients most needed for immune efficiency and using therapeutic intervention to reduce viral and other infections and to correct allergic conditions if this is needed.)

Coping Skills

Dr Clive Wood of the Department of Human Sciences at Oxford University has shown ('Are Happy People Healthier?' *Journal of the Royal Society of Medicine*, June 1987) that physical health and immune function are enhanced if a constellation of attitudes can be influenced so that what is known as the 'hardiness' factor is developed.

Specific biochemical changes are observed in people with feelings of helplessness in the face of the perceived threats of life. These changes result in reduced immune efficiency. Conversely, development of 'hardiness' has the effect of restoring immune efficiency, when faced by the same threats and stresses.

Hardiness is defined as an element, inborn in many people but which can be learned by others, which consists of three components:

1 *The control factor*, which involves a sense of control over one's environment. People with this feeling of control act and function in a manner which indicates that they, and not others, or their environment, govern what they will do and what happens in life. They do not feel 'buffeted by fate' but in control of their destiny.

2 *The commitment factor*, which relates to the degree of our involvement in life, as evidenced by the degree of interest and curiosity we show and the interaction we enjoy with people and society.

3 *The challenge factor*, which is characterized by having expectations of impending change and the future not as threats or burdens, but rather as positive challenges which will be met and overcome, leading naturally to personal growth and development.

As Dr Wood puts it, 'Several studies have shown that possession of the "hardy" personality buffers the effects of a stressful environment and results in less frequent and less severe ill-health among groups with high, as opposed to low, levels of hardiness.' An optimistic appraisal of events in life, and a tendency to take decisive rather than evasive action in response to these, is the heart of 'hardiness'.

It is known that by careful and diligent application we can train ourselves to adopt the elements which make up hardiness, thus reaping the health benefits which it bestows.

This may call for counselling for some people, although self-administered change is also possible by the simple expedient of practising, at every opportunity, what are seen to be the desirable characteristics of hardiness (accepting responsibility for what happens, positive attitude, active decision-making in response to events, optimism, involvement in life, feelings of 'Looking on the bright side' etc.) and avoiding habitual 'non-hardiness' behaviour (avoidance of responsibility for what happens, negativity, passivity, pessimism, non-involvement in life, feelings of 'If something can go wrong for me it will,' etc.).

Far from being peripheral to the problem of ill-health in general, and susceptibility to infection in particular (and therefore to ME) this concept of personality and stress-coping skills is a central and vital factor. There is no guilt or blame attached to the possession of a particular set of attitudes and behaviour patterns. These were inborn or acquired in early life. But they can be changed, if you can recognize the usefulness of such change.

It may be that some professional guidance would be required, and this should not be avoided. The very grasping of the nettle can be the first and most important step in showing that there is no longer need to fear, that things can only improve if you open yourself to change and to growth.

Fact and Fantasy

Apart from the habits of personality with which we are equipped, many of us also carry a potentially harmful pattern of behaviour. This relates to a failure to differentiate easily between the reality of our life and personal environment (work, family, economics, relationships etc.), and these same elements as we fantasize or imagine they ought to be.

It has been suggested by psychotherapists and workers in the area of stress-management that in essence emotional stress arises as a direct result of a failure on our part to reconcile reality with our fantasy of how things should be.

If I believe that a person ought to behave in a particular way and they do not do so, this creates stress, whether this is something related to work, family or the general interaction in daily life with others. I may become angry, edgy, moody, or in some other way show that things are not as I would like them to be or as I believe they should be. This harms me. I could on the other hand explain to the person my feelings, in a non-belligerent and concise way, and call for altered behaviour, which may or may not be forthcoming. This would represent my attempt to alter the factors which I do not like.

If the desired changes are forthcoming (my neighbour stops playing his transistor radio full blast in the garden, my wife stops wearing her hair in curlers all day, my child stops calling me 'Pops' etc. etc.) then I will have successfully dealt with a potential source of stress. I will have exerted the 'control' factor and altered my environment.

If no good response is forthcoming I will at least have expressed myself rather than holding the problem inside myself. Expressing feelings reduces the stress element, at least somewhat. Or I might have to take other action. This could involve altering my attitude to the perceived stress. I can try to get to like the music which I cannot escape from or learn not to hear it by practising meditation techniques (see below), or wear ear plugs or move house. These actions involve personal accommodation to something which apparently cannot be changed. This reduces stress just as effectively as any change I might engineer in the 'problem'. I change myself or my attitude and therefore the problem is no longer so pressing. The direct evasion of wearing ear plugs, moving home or calling the police represent further attempts to change the environment, variations on the theme of 'control'.

These examples illustrate the possibilities which exist in all problems for action other than worrying, fretting, brooding etc. If we analyse the situation we can see that reality (the loud music) and my fantasy (peace) do not match. Either I alter reality or I alter my fantasy, if I wish to avoid self-destructive emotions from operating inside me.

In relation to more serious life events, job-loss, bereavement, financial crisis etc. we have similar choices. We can do all that is practically feasible in situations where some action is possible, or we can accept reality where nothing is possible in terms of changing the facts. We can learn to think along lines which say, 'Since there is no choice, since it has happened, since I cannot alter it, I accept it and now move on to areas I can do something about.'

This does not mean liking what has happened or is about to happen. It means recognizing that anything other than such an attitude (of accepting what cannot be changed) is self-destructive, and that such behaviour is not in our best interests.

The same life event faced by different people produces different responses. Following a disaster or crisis in your life, a degree of depression is normal. However, if it is inordinately prolonged, the reaction becomes health- and life-threatening. In such a case there is frequently a failure or inability to accept the reality of what has happened. Often there is a tendency towards thoughts of 'If only' or 'Why?' and not an attempt to accept the inevitable and to carry on with the multitude of things that can and need to be done.

Without labouring this too much, it is necessary, if anxiety and worry are major elements in your life, to look at whether you are accepting (or trying to change) 'what is' or whether you are living with a great deal of 'if only' and doing little to bring reality and fantasy together.

This is not a prescription for defeatism. Rather, it is a call for positive action where this is possible – including expressing to those who matter the feelings which lie behind the desire for changes – or for a recognition that it will be beneficial to alter attitudes and behaviour patterns in order to take account of what cannot be changed. These strategies help prevent negative emotional and life-damaging reactions in the immune system. It is not stress which damages us, it is our response to stress.

Relaxing and Stretching Tight Tense Muscles

We tense muscles in response to stress and anxiety. If the tension is of anything but short duration, the muscular changes which occur become semi-permanent as muscles shorten and lay down supporting fibres to maintain the tension. This is enormously wasteful of energy, and leads not only to stiffness and perhaps pain but to tiredness and reduced functional ability.

If, as is all too common, the muscles of the neck, shoulders, upper chest and diaphragm region are involved, the efficiency of the breathing function can be seriously impaired, encouraging incorrect muscular action, poor rib excursion and hyperventilation.

A truism in osteopathy is that function (the way something works) is directly and totally interrelated with its structure (the way it is made). If structural changes occur and muscles become short, tense and tight they cannot function as they would if they were loose, elastic and free. This loss of functional ability, especially in relation to breathing, is very important to the person with ME as it impinges on the ability to obtain enough oxygen through full respiration, as well as increasing the likelihood of hyperventilation (over-breathing) as the body attempts to obtain enough oxygen via its faulty machinery.

Energy conservation and the ability to get enough oxygen to meet requirements without creating chemical imbalances through hyperventilation, call for the relaxation and stretching of any tense short muscles and the mobilizing of restricted joints resulting from these muscular changes, followed by the re-learning of good breathing habits.

Treatment involving deep soft-tissue manipulation, massage and osteopathic or chiropractic manipulation may be called for in order to achieve the first goal of normalized structure. If the rib-cage and upper spinal region are very tense this needs to be dealt with before breathing exercises can be effectively performed, since trying to use the breathing apparatus before it is adequately free is self-defeating.

If muscular tension is not too chronic it is possible, through breathing exercises and self-administered stretching (yoga-type) movements, to restore a good deal of normality to respiration.

We must not lose sight of the fact that those with ME are limited in what they can or should do at any one time in terms of muscular effort. I have found that gentle stretching exercises are acceptable in most cases of ME, if the pattern of little and often is followed and no heroic efforts are made.

Before stretching proper is attempted, however, the muscles need to be relaxed, and the safest method for the person with ME is a form of modified autogenic training.

Autogenic Training

A.T. instruction is available from teachers in many parts of Britain. It is being used very successfully by British GP Kai Kermani for people with AIDS. The method incorporates deep relaxation with specific techniques which can draw out painful emotions. Most of the nearly one hundred people with AIDS who have been through Dr Kermani's autogenic workshops have outlasted conventional life expectancy, many in apparently good health despite having full-blown AIDS.

This is of some importance to people with ME since if a battered immune system can be helped to function again, one which is only slightly dented should do significantly better.

The value of A.T. as opposed to most other forms of muscular relaxation for people with ME is highlighted by a correspondent in New Zealand, writing to the Journal of the Australian and New Zealand ME Society (May 1986). She says, 'I tried various relaxing programmes but none of them helped. They all seemed to begin "Now tense such-and-such a muscle". For ME and me the last thing that did any good was tensing a muscle.' She continues, 'When I got the ANZMES relaxation tape I found to my relief that there was an alternative method of relaxing.'

Autogenic training, which was developed in Canada and is now used worldwide, does not demand the initial tensing of muscles that is a feature of progressive muscular relaxation. It asks instead that you focus your mind on one part of your body at a time, and that you mentally visualize, or instruct it to feel, either warm or heavy.

It has been shown that if a body thermometer is attached to the hand and this technique is then applied ('My hand is feeling – or getting – warm[er]') for a minute or so, the temperature actually rises. This happens because as muscular tension reduces, the circulation to the part improves, warming it significantly.

You may not actually sense any change in warmth or feelings of heaviness as you do the exercise; on the other hand you may. It really does not matter a great deal. What does matter is that you are learning to focus on one area and function at a time, thus stilling the incessant chatter of thoughts which most of us have as a constant element in our minds. This starts the relaxation process. More than this is happening though, most importantly a release of long-held tensions in the muscles. A by-product is that local circulation will improve.

A.T. should be learned from a teacher. If this is not possible then the shortened or modified method which is described below can be used.

Modified A.T. Exercise

Start by lying comfortably on the floor with a pillow under the head, knees bent or resting over a cushion to release tension in the low back. You should be warm but not hot and should ensure that none of your clothing is tight and that there are no distracting sounds at the time. This is best done some time after a meal, say mid-morning or mid-afternoon, or last thing at night.

In order to enhance relaxation and actually modify the brain-wave rhythms in such a way as to induce a meditative or hypnotic state, you should roll your eyeballs (closed eyes) upwards and slightly inwards, as though you were looking 'at the centre of the forehead'. This has been shown to produce a desirable neurophysiological change which makes the subsequent exercise more efficient. *This should be done whenever you induce visualization (see below).*

Focus your mind on your dominant arm (right arm if you are right-handed) and say to yourself (in your mind), 'My right hand (or arm) is feeling warm.' This statement is followed by some seconds (10 to 20) of 'watching' or sensing the feelings in the arm. You may try to imagine that the arm is having sunlight shining on it, or that it is being warmed by a fire. Sensations of warmth or tingling may or may not be felt. Repeat the statement several times with pauses for focusing on the arm or hand.

Now do the same thing with the other arm (hand). Then progressively work around the body, going to the left leg and then the right leg, following the same sequence of making the statement several times then allowing a pause for observation of subjective feelings. There will be a natural tendency to lose concentration, for your mind to wander off into thoughts and daydreams. Do not let this worry you. Simply return to the pattern where you left off.

Having performed the 'warming' exercise on the four limbs, return to the first place of attention, the right arm, and this time instead of stating to it that it feels warm(er) tell it that it is feeling heavy.

A sensation of the limb being leaden, an immovable deadweight, is what you are seeking. Do not do anything consciously such as pushing it down against the floor. Simply make the statement and observe this sensation. It may or may not be something you are aware of. Repeat this several times before moving on to the other arm and then to first one and then the other leg, going through the same sequence with each.

Finish the exercise by concentrating on your forehead, accompanied by a statement of 'my head is feeling cool'. As you make this statement try to visualize a cool breeze playing on your head. Repeat this statement and observation several times before luxuriating for some minutes in a sense of overall relaxation, stillness, heaviness, peace and well-being.

Conclude with the statement 'I am alert and refreshed'. You may well fall asleep before coming to the end of the exercise, and you will almost certainly lose concentration many times at first. It helps some people to record the 'statements' on to a tape, with appropriate lengths of pause between, thus allowing all the attention to be focused on whatever sensations are apparent. Try this if you find the mental instruction process cumbersome.

Full autogenic training concentrates attention on breathing and heart function as well. However, for the purposes of beginning to learn relaxation this modified method has proved very successful. You should work through the sequence at least once every day and should take not less than 10 and not more than 20 minutes to perform adequately.

Relieving Muscle Pain and Muscle Tightness

When muscles are painful they tighten and when muscles are tight they become painful. In the event of short-term strains and stresses this state of affairs usually passes on its own. However when it is prolonged and chronic, physical changes occur in the soft tissues which require treatment (often self-applied) in order to stretch what has become tight or to remove focal points of irritation, known as trigger points, which generate pain. If your back muscles in general are stiff and tight, with no particular pathology of the joints creating the problem but rather as a result of inactivity or over-use, stretching would probably relieve them.

In ME the build-up of lactic acid in the muscles is very similar to the situation which occurs when excessive exercise has been performed in 'normal' people. Stretching allows for freer circulation and for 'flushing' of these acids from the muscles. In the case of ME this would only be of temporary benefit but should nonetheless be welcome and relieving.

There are two basic principles which we can use to allow muscles to be stretched easily, without undue effort. These are Post-Isometric Relaxation (PIR) and Reciprocal Inhibition (RI).

How to Use PIR and RI

Let us return to the example of the stiff back muscles. If you were to bend forwards (sitting in a chair or standing) you would reach a 'barrier' preventing further bending, which is set for you by the tight muscles. If at this point you were

140

to try to return to the upright position (using only a small part of the strength of the muscles of the back) but were gently prevented from doing so by the restraining hands of someone else, for about 10 seconds, something unexpected would happen.

When you ceased the attempt to sit upright, and the friend/helper ceased restraining you, the tight muscles would be obliged to relax because of a phenomenon known as Post-Isometric Relaxation. When a muscle tries to move and is prevented from doing so by an equal and opposite force PIR results immediately after the effort.

It is now well established that the effort required need only be minimal and should not involve heroic pushing or pulling. Once the isometric effort (equal but opposite forces preventing motion during effort) is released the bend forwards would then go further than was previously possible, without any effort, because of the release of tension in these muscles, which is automatic after such an effort.

This principle can be used to help the release and relaxation of any stiff muscles or joints. It is usual to perform the same gentle isometric effort several times (starting from the new 'barrier' since you will now be able to bend further) until no more release is forthcoming.

Exactly the opposite direction of effort (if restrained) produces a similar effect for different reasons. Imagine that you were to bend forwards as far as was comfortable and that at that point you were restrained from bending further forwards by someone standing behind you and passing their hands around your abdomen. The muscles in the front of the body would be trying to take you forwards but would be being isometrically restricted from doing so.

If this was a gentle, 7 to 10 second, effort (using only about 10 or 15 per cent of the available energy in the muscle, which is probably all anyone with ME could manage without excessively tiring themselves) another remarkable effect would be produced. On release of the effort to bend forwards, and of the counter-effort which was restraining it, the muscles of the back which were tight would have released somewhat because of reciprocal inhibition.

Why is this? All muscles have antagonists which release and relax as their opposite number, the agonist, tightens to perform a task, thus allowing smooth, co-ordinated movements. When an antagonist is isometrically contracted the agonist relaxes automatically. When the abdominal muscles try to bend you forward and are prevented from doing so by the restraining hands of your helper, the back muscles have to relax. After this you can bend forwards more easily.

These principles can be applied to any stiff joint or tight muscle. Use minimal effort and maintain this for 7 to 10 seconds using either the stiff muscles themselves or their antagonists, always gently restrained from actually moving.

In some instances a helper is not needed and an immovable object can be used for the counter-effort. If opening the fingers of the hand is difficult because of joint or muscle restriction then trying to open the fingers against resistance provided by your other hand will produce PIR. Trying to close the stiff fingers against resistance provided by a hard ball (for example) would produce RI.

It may be easier to grasp these ideas if you think of the barrier, the point of limitation or the direction in which it is difficult to move a part (hand, elbow, back, neck etc.). If you take the area (joint, muscle, region etc.) to that barrier of resistance, without effort or strain, and then, against resistance, try either to go through the barrier (therefore using antagonists to the tight muscles) or come away from the barrier (using the short muscles themselves) you will achieve one or other of these two possibilities, RI or PIR.

142

Trigger Points

If there exists muscular pain, or pain in a general area which involves soft tissues, you can establish immediately whether or not that pain is locally generated or is a referred pain coming from a distant 'trigger' point.

Press on the painful area. Does the pain increase? If so the pain is locally generated. If on pressing a painful region no increase in pain is felt, then almost certainly the pain being felt is coming from a reference area somewhere else in the body.

Such trigger points are local areas of extremely powerful neurological activity which influence the local nerves and which pass messages via the central nervous system to other regions, creating pain and other symptoms. If you find, by careful prodding and squeezing, a local area in a muscle which not only feels very sensitive itself, but which is also hard and knotted, and which after a few seconds of maintained pressure sends painful impulses to a distant part of the body, you have found a trigger point.

There are many of these to be found in tight muscles anywhere in the body, especially the neck and shoulder region from which trigger points often send their aberrant pain impulses to the head or face, or into the arms. The scope of this book does not allow for a full description of how to deal with these, although self-treatment is usually possible, involving as it does pressure applied to the trigger, followed by chilling the region (using ice or special cold sprays) and then stretching the affected muscle (using the methods described above).

I suggest that anyone who wishes to use these methods on themselves or their friends (they are completely safe if the basic rules are followed) read my book *Instant Pain Control* (Thorsons 1983) which is designed for the lay reader. A fuller explanation designed for the professional therapist is to be found in another of my books, *Soft Tissue*

Manipulation (Thorsons 1987), which also provides detailed descriptions of the use of PIR and RI (collectively known as 'muscle energy techniques').

People with ME have a need to try *gently* to deal with the muscular aspects of their problem, using methods which do not tire them further. Removal of trigger points is important in preserving energy that is being wastefully used by these chaotic muscular bundles, which produce pain and discomfort which further drains already limited energy supplies.

A visit to a competent osteopath, chiropractor, physiotherapist or massage therapist who deals with the soft-tissue structures (not all manipulative therapists are prepared to deal with this most vital area) is an excellent way of assisting with such problems. Treatment using acupuncture is another very effective method of removing trigger points and is recommended for everyone with ME. This is discussed in more detail in Chapter 12.

Prolonged Respiratory Exhalation as a Means of Reducing Arousal

It is my belief that before attempting to learn breathing techniques an assessment and appropriate treatment from an osteopath, chiropractor or physiotherapist is desirable so that structural factors preventing good respiration can be dealt with first.

There is however one technique which is particularly relevant to people with ME, and which can be learned irrespective of the functional ability of the breathing mechanisms. Ancient yoga breathing methods have recently been researched in American university settings with quite remarkable results.

Different patterns of breathing were used by volunteers in the face of threatened pain and during various emotionally stressful situations. Only one pattern of breathing was consistently found to reduce the degree of arousal which such stresses normally produce (so effectively keeping the person more relaxed). There were a variety of measurements taken during these studies including that of skin resistance to electricity, a standard means of assessing whether a person is reacting to stress. (Skin resistance rises as we relax and falls as we become anxious.)

The method which worked in all situations of physical and mental stress was one which can be practised by anyone with perfect safety. Bruce Cappo and David Holmes concluded their report on the research, 'The results of this investigation provide consistent evidence that rapid inhalation followed by slow exhalation in an overall pattern of reduced respiration rate can be an effective technique for reducing physiological and psychological arousal when anticipating and confronting threat. The technique has been advocated by yogi masters for many years, but this appears to be the first controlled test of its utility.'

The method calls firstly for a *slowing down* of the overall rate of breathing to 6 cycles per minute. This means that each full cycle should take 10 seconds (for a complete cycle of breathing in and breathing out). The next demand is that the exhalation phase should take significantly longer than the inhalation phase. Ideally in healthy volunteers this led to a 2 second breathing-in phase followed by a very slow 8 second breathing-out phase. In practice this may not be too easy for anyone who is not fit at the outset, although it should be the pattern to aim for.

To start the practice sessions, have a watch with a second-hand sweep easily visible and try to breathe in fully in not more than 4 seconds. Immediately start to exhale and take a full 6 seconds to do so (if the inhalation was 4 seconds that is – if it took 3 seconds to breathe in then exhale for 7 seconds). Practice this sequence of swift inhalation and slow exhalation for a 5 minute period at least once a day.

After a few weeks you will have the timing off pat and will probably no longer need the watch to assist your cycles. As time goes by you will also find that you can get closer to the 2 seconds in, 8 seconds out, pattern which the yogi masters and the American researchers advocate.

After any such training session you may feel light-headed. Rest for some minutes with no particular breathing control and normality will return. Only use the technique in daily life when you feel stressed, angered, aroused, anxious or threatened, and it will calm you and prevent you from going into a hyperventilation pattern of breathing. Heightened arousal and hyperventilation is a factor in some but not all people with ME, but knowledge of correct breathing is of value in all conditions.

Other Breathing Techniques

Once you have had your thoracic mechanics assessed and suitably normalized by treatment you can begin to learn to use your breathing equipment correctly. This involves learning diaphragmatic (abdominal) breathing as well as lateral chest breathing methods in various positions – lying, sitting and standing.

In any (and all) of these positions rest your hands on the area between the lower ribs and your navel and as you start to breathe in (through the nose ideally) try consciously to push this region outwards (so that if you are lying down your hands will be pushed towards the ceiling) and fill the lower lungs with the breath. This inhalation should take 3 to 4 seconds and should be followed by a slow exhalation which takes slightly longer than the inhalation.

Again you are trying to slow down the overall rhythm of breathing to no more than 8 or 9 cycles per minute during the exercise. This pattern of inhalation (one, two, three, four) pause, exhalation (one, two, three, four, five) is repeated 5 or 6 times at first, rising ultimately, as the muscles and energy levels allow it, to 15 to 20 times.

Gradually you should find that the abdominal expansion (which allows the diaphragm to descend) becomes less of a conscious effort and more of an automatic process. The timing will also become automatic.

After the abdominal phase, place your hands on the lower ribs with the tips of the fingers facing forwards. Breathe to the same rhythm, but this time instead of pushing the abdomen forwards as you inhale try to force the hands apart as the lower ribs expand sideways. As you exhale again allow these ribs to 'collapse' together as the hands come together. Use a slight push with the hands to ensure that you have breathed out fully before the next inhalation commences. Again do this 5 or 6 times at first and gradually increase the number of repetitions as energy and stamina allows.

This pattern of breathing will also reduce the chances of hyperventilation if applied in stressful conditions.

Mind Power

You should learn, too, a method of meditation. This can be done from tapes, books or teachers. There are numerous methods and not all will suit each of us. Somewhere in the range of available methods will be one which is best suited to your make-up and mental state. I have described a number of meditation methods in my book *Your Complete Stress-Proofing Programme* (Thorsons 1986).

Once you have learned to relax physically (the autogenic method above) you are half-way to effective meditation, which involves use of 'something' (a sound, an idea, an image, a word etc.) to focus on, and which effectively stills the mind and allows healing to progress more rapidly.

Once you have been able to so still the mind (and the autogenic method can often do this too, as well as more mentally directed meditations) you are ready for guided imagery or visualization techniques. This ultimately calls for you to visualize a desired healing process and mentally to encourage this. (The most dramatic evidence of the effectiveness of such methods has come in conditions like cancer and AIDS. Books such as *Getting Well Again* by Dr Carl Simonton and his wife Stephanie Mathews-Simonton (1980) as well as *Mind as Healer, Mind as Slayer* by Kenneth Pelletier (1977) document the amazing power of healing which the mind possesses.)

In order to embark on visualization, then, there is a need first to quiet the mind's babble and chatter and to learn how to focus it. This is why the process of relaxation (autogenic in this case) followed by meditation is suggested before the guided imagery (visualization methods) are attempted. Initially a general exercise is suggested to begin the process of exercising the potential of the mind.

'Safe Haven' Exercise

After your autogenic training has been practised for some weeks you should be beginning to experience something close to relaxation. Now, at the end of the exercise spend a minute doing the following exercise.

Imagine a real or fictitious place in which you would be happy, safe and content. You may have the sort of imagination which allows for such a picture to be visualized (as though on a screen) or you may only be able to imagine it in some other way. Let us say the picture of your safe place (safe haven) is a room. It may be a pleasant panelled room with a fireplace and comfortable armchairs, lovely curtains and pictures. Try to 'see' these details. Try to hear the crackle of the fire, the music from the radio etc. Try to smell the flowers in the vase on the table and to feel the softness of the chair on which you are sitting. See also other people if you wish to, enjoying this lovely room. In other words use all your senses in this exercise. You are not only seeing things but trying to make them more real by smelling and feeling and hearing them as well.

Spend a minute or two in this scene and when you leave it know that you can go back any time, and that since it is your fantasy you can change anything you wish. You may also want at another time to try to visualize something quite different, say a garden scene or being by the seaside or by a river. Again, use all your senses to bring in colours, odours and sounds.

Repeat this exercise after each relaxation session or whenever you feel a desire to escape into a beautiful scene. Its purpose is to sharpen your imaginative powers, which you will then use for more practical purposes in your healing process.

Guided Imagery in Healing

When you have spent some weeks using your safe haven you can begin to use the imaginative powers of the mind to direct aspects of the healing process. If it is energy that is your main concern you might, after appropriate relaxation, direct attention towards the way your body makes and uses energy. This can be quite 'scientific' if you have a know-ledge of the process, or it can be completely 'comic book' imagery if you have only a vague idea of the processes involved.

In dealing with cancer the Simontons found that some people were able to see clearly the defence mechanisms acting against tumour cells and to visualize the successful completion of such events. Other people had no detailed awareness of how these internal battles took place and visualized their white (defending) blood cells as knights in armour and the tumour cells as grey slug-like enemies which the victorious knights demolished in battle.

Dr Simonton was an orthodox medical specialist using radiotherapy to treat cancer. He observed that some of his patients did better than others and that those who were most responsive had a more positive will to live and a more hopeful attitude towards the therapy they were receiving. After studying a number of techniques, including autogenic training, Simonton developed the technique of relaxation followed by positive imagery, which he taught to all of his patients. He asked his patients in their imagery to visualize the way their body was interacting with the therapy they were receiving, and to see their tumours vanishing. The results were astounding. The more co-operative and positive the patient, the better the results. The deeper the relaxation achieved, the better the results.

Hope and positive imagery are powerful healing tools and we can harness them if we release scepticism and doubt. You have nothing to lose but your illness.

In a book on AIDS which I co-authored with Simon Martin, we describe how a skin lesion known as kaposi's sarcoma was dealt with by one person with AIDS who visualized this and then 'saw' a rubber erasing the blemish in his mind. Objective improvement took place after this imagery.

A far more remarkable piece of evidence for the use of imagery is also cited in the same book. This relates to Jay Baldwin, a nurse from San Francisco with AIDS, who learned to visualize his white blood cells being manufactured, to great advantage. At one point in his saga he was hospitalized with gram-negative shock when his white blood count dropped to 600. He refused various medical procedures since he knew from experience that in his current state he would probably not survive them, but after intense visualization his white blood count went up to 11,600 in 36 hours. The doctors who came in with the results refused to believe that both the specimen from the emergency room and the specimen taken 36 hours later could both be Baldwin's blood. At Baldwin's insistence, further tests were done to establish that both specimens were indeed his own blood. At three in the morning the doctor came back and confirmed that they were. Baldwin was back at work within a week.

Jay Baldwin had an advantage in knowing precisely where and how his white blood cells were made and he could use this in his visualization, but use of non-scientific imagery is often equally effective in enhancing the healing process.

Imagery for ME

The type of imagery that helps you will depend upon which elements are most active in the production of your ME.

If allergies and sensitivities are involved, then visualizing your immune system dealing normally with current allergens (from food, or inhaled) with no untoward reaction would be a positive aid to this happening.

If candida is active you might try a visualization exercise in which you 'see' the various therapeutic efforts you are making (taking acidophilus – friendly bacteria – using antifungal substances and nutrients, removing those foods the yeast loves such as sugar etc.) starving the fungus, and your immune system becoming activated to remove the overgrowth from regions in which it does not belong.

If exhaustion is the major symptom you might try to visualize energy-production being enhanced, and this new-found energy flooding through the system, energizing the muscles and your brain. Your image could include a happy, healthy and active you, doing things in which you are at present limited by the condition.

If pain and stiffness are current, use the visualization method to see the pain vanish, to feel the stiffness release and to imagine yourself active, energetic and pain-free.

Whatever aspect of your condition requires your attention, address this in visualization, seeing the changes you wish to take place happening, using accurate or totally fanciful images, whichever make more sense to you. The body responds either way.

Were it not for people such as the Simontons who have used these techniques for over ten years in people with cancer, and for the many people with AIDS who have used visualization to remarkable effect in checking deterioration and actually coming back to reasonable levels of health, you would be forgiven for scepticism about this approach.

But the method works, and its limitations appear to be created only by the mind of the person using it. If you *know* that visualization and your mind can not only slightly influence, but can actually control, most of the processes going on inside you (good and bad) you can use it to dramatic purpose.

REFERENCES

A Gentle Way with Cancer, Kidman, B., Century, London 1983.
'Anxiety and Muscle Tension Pain', Barlow, W., *British Journal of Clinical Practice*, vol. 13, no. 5, pp. 339–49, 1959.
A World without AIDS, Chaitow, L., Martin, S., Thorsons, Wellingborough 1988.
'Enhanced Adaptive Response in Patients Pretreated with Breathing Retraining', Bonn, J., Readhead, C., *The Lancet*, 22 September 1984, pp. 665–9.
Getting Well Again, Simonton, C. and S., Bantam Books, London 1980.
Instant Pain Control, Chaitow, L., Thorsons, Wellingborough 1983.

Mind as Healer, Mind as Slayer, Pelletier, K., Delta, New York 1977.
'Utility of Prolonged Respiratory Exhalation for Reducing Arousal', Cappo, B., Holmes, D., *Journal of Psychosomatic Research*, vol. 28, no. 4, pp. 265–73, 1984.
Your Complete Stress-Proofing Programme, Chaitow, L., Thorsons, Wellingborough 1985.

11 Antiviral Methods

The virus is not the cause of any disease. It may play a very real role in ME or any other infection, but it can only thrive, replicate and cause ill-health if the immune system of the person it is infecting is unable to control it. The soil in which the virus grows is therefore where our primary therapeutic effort should always be directed.

Such efforts towards enhancement of the immune system form the major elements in my suggested approach to the problem of ME and any persistent viral activity, however intermittent this may be.

Medical science knows of very few effective antiviral substances which are not themselves highly toxic. There are, however, several 'alternative' methods, substances and approaches which have proven antiviral potentials. It is these which I shall describe below.

Lysine and Herpes Viruses

We have already seen that an approach using the amino acid lysine is capable of slowing the multiplication and activity of the herpes family of viruses of which Epstein-

Barr is one. I have described this in Chapter 9 because it is a purely nutritional method, using a strategy of increasing dietary lysine levels by eating foods rich in this amino acid, as well as taking lysine supplementation, at the same time as reducing arginine-rich foods in the diet.

If any of the herpes viruses are implicated in your condition this is a primary and effective approach.

AL721

Another (almost) nutritional approach involves the use of a number of lipid (fatty) substances mainly derived from egg yolk lecithin.

In the late 1970s a team of researchers under Dr Meir Shinitsky, at the Weizmann Institute in Israel, developed a formulation for a mixture of lipids extracted from egg yolks and blended with neutral fats (such as butter) which was named AL721. AL stands for 'active lecithin' and the 721 stands for the ratio between the neutral lipids (7 parts) and phosphatidylcholine (pure lecithin – 2 parts) and phosphatidylethanolamine (a part of lecithin – 1 part).

This formula was initially used in treating aspects of cancer, where it was shown to have an immune-enhancing effect (it was also found to be useful in cases of impaired memory and when treating people withdrawing from drugs). The scientific rationale for its use can be found in a two-volume study by Dr Shinitsky entitled *Physiology of Membrane Fluidity* (1984).

Excitement was generated amongst people with AIDS when, in 1985, AL721 was cited in the *New England Journal of Medicine* by no less an authority than Dr Robert Gallo as being worthy of serious research, since in laboratory conditions it had been shown to prevent human T-cells from becoming infected by HIV, the purported AIDS virus.

Since that time a veritable industry has grown around the 'underground' manufacture of AL721 'look-alike' products because AL721 itself was only slowly moving through the laborious process of acquiring a product licence from the authorities in the USA. Many AIDS patients who have had AL721 treatment have reported remarkable benefits. This is documented in my book (co-authored with Simon Martin) *A World without AIDS* (Thorsons 1988).

A commercially produced 'clone' of AL721 is available in the UK under the name of VM1, and many people have, as well, put together the basic ingredients in their kitchen blenders (recipe and contact number for VM1 below).

How Can Active Lecithin Affect Viral Activity?

AL721 is thought to be the first of a class of medicines which modify cell membranes to achieve treatment goals. 'Membrane engineering' in this instance increases what is called the 'micro-fluidity' of the cell membranes, thus making it more difficult for viruses to attach to receptor sites and so enter and infect the cell.

It is also thought that AL721 removes cholesterol-like substances from the envelope which surrounds the virus, thus further interfering with important receptor configurations and rendering the virus less infectious. According to John James, editor of *AIDS Treatment News*: 'Theory suggests that in addition to AIDS *AL721 might also help against other lipid-coated viruses such as herpes, cytomegalovirus and Epstein-Barr. It was found to be effective against herpes in one animal study, reported in October 1986 at a symposium in New Orleans* [my italics].' It is the lipid (fatty) protective coat, which characterizes the herpes family of viruses, which seems to be what allows AL721 effectively to deactivate them.

Only a few clinical studies have so far been reported

(there are hundreds of individual testimonials and anec-dotal reports of its usefulness). One, conducted at St Luke's Roosevelt Hospital, New York City, showed a remarkable 80 to 90 per cent drop in HIV activity in five of seven patients with AIDS treated with AL721, and in some of these no HIV activity at all could be found after just two weeks on the substance.

In Tel Aviv, Israel, Dr Yahuda Skornik has treated many people with AIDS using AL721. In October 1987 he revealed that of 60 patients treated thus far in that year, 58 were showing improvement. Several of his patients had been very advanced at the start, and some who were considered terminal had had their conditions reversed and were improving in health. Of those taking AL721 for 5 months or more, platelet levels in the blood improved in all of them, in one case going from 16,000 to 110,000 in a month. In most the white blood counts improved consistently.

In the UK the DHSS is aware of these studies but no large follow-up trials have so far been conducted. In July 1988 Mr Peter Rost MP (Erewash), at the behest of the *Journal of Alternative and Complementary Medicine*, asked the Minister of Health, the Rt. Hon. Tony Newton MP, whether there had been any trial of the formulation AL721 (active lecithin).

The reply he received was: 'We are not aware of any research being funded in this area. I am advised that in individual cases of AIDS there may be a need for specific nutritional supplementation, but for the generality of cases there is no evidence that anything other than a good balanced diet is required.' The minister went on to say that for reasons of commercial confidentiality he was unable to comment on whether any manufacturer had applied for a product licence or clinical trial certificate for lecithin or any other potential treatment for AIDS.

Since we are talking about butter and eggs blended together in specific ratios it is hard to see why something reportedly of marked benefit to people with persistent viral infections should require complex trials. *There is nothing to prevent anyone with ME from using AL721 if they can obtain it, or its clone VM1 which is easily available, if they have any evidence of persistent or recurrent viral activity especially related to herpes viruses (Epstein-Barr, cytomegalovirus, herpes simplex etc.).* AL721 is totally non-toxic. It is refrigerated and before use is spread on bread just like butter, and is then eaten.

Do-It-Yourself AL721 Substitute

John James who publishes the *AIDS Treatment News* in San Francisco has given the recipe for making a substitute for AL721 in your kitchen.

You will need to obtain egg yolk lecithin (soya doesn't work as well) in the correct balance of 2 parts phosphatidylcholine to 1 part phosphatidylethanolamine. This can be purchased as PC55 from Twin Laboratories Ltd, Ronkonkoma, New York. All you then need is a blender and some butter.

Recipe (With thanks to John James for this *approximation* of AL721)

1 Combine 5 tablespoons of PC55 and 12 tablespoons of water and whip in a blender/mixer.
2 Measure out 6 tablespoons plus one teaspoon of butter and melt it before adding to the water/PC55 mixture and again blending briskly for 3 to 5 minutes.
3 Divide the resulting mixture into 10 equal portions (each will weigh around 1.06 ounces/30.4 grams). It is a good idea to place individual doses in separate plastic bags.
4 Freeze these immediately as the mixture spoils quickly. Remove individual doses from the freezer *to*

the refrigerator a few hours before use and take two doses daily spread on bread or mixed in juice, and avoid consuming any other fat at that time.

I would stress to you that this kitchen-made approximation of AL721 is not the same as the original, which requires some technical wizardry to achieve the ideal blend and ratio. However it does have antiviral potential for any of the lipid-coated viruses, most of which have been associated w''ı ME.

Note also that there have been reports of virus 'rebound' if AL721 is taken and suddenly stopped. Keep going for a considerable time once you start.

A clone of AL721 is VM1 and a phone call to 01 (London) 299-1409 will put you in touch with a supply of this.

Italian Antiviral Medication

Italian research and clinical practice have produced a potentially very useful means of stopping viral activity in a non-toxic manner. This requires the injection by a doctor of very small amounts of a medication which is, or was, commonly used in large doses in treating amoebic dysentery, namely emetine hydrochloride.

This application of what has long been a medication in use for control of amoebic infections outside the intestine, as well as in treating amoebic dysentery, is based on the work of the late Dr Antonio Fusillo of Bari, Italy. The information which I have included below derives mainly from Dr Fusillo's report which was presented to a group in Bari a few years ago (the paper, entitled 'Prospects of a New Anti-Viral Chemotherapy', is undated, but contains references as recent as 1983).

The report discusses over twenty years of work conducted by Italian researchers (named as Professors B. Loddo, P. La Colla, G. Cocuzza, A. San Filippo) into antiviral

chemotherapy, the results of which were presented in
October 1980 at the 2nd Covegno Nazionale di Roma
(published in *Atti*, vol. 1, Relazioni, page 385) and which
stated that emetine has, 'The capacity to act against virus
DNA and RNA.'

Dr Fusillo tells us that he began use of emetine hydrochloride in 1963 when he treated dogs with amoebic
dysentery. He discovered that its well known toxic effects
when given in high doses were absent when used in very
small doses. He used rabbits for further study since they are
noted to be extremely sensitive to emetine.

He showed, in one trial, that three rabbits survived
through the use of minute amounts of emetine hydrochloride, after being inoculated with 5 cc of brain extract
derived from a rabid dog (provided by the director of the
Istituto di Zooprofilassi di Portici).

In human trials he first demonstrated emetine's rapid
and safe effects in cases of herpes zoster (shingles). Use of 2
to 3 milligrams of emetine HC1, by injection under the skin,
produced rapid healing, including an end to the violent
pain within two to three days of its use. This benefit was
shown to be produced in repeated instances of herpes
zoster.

A colleague, Professor Quesada, showed outstanding
antiviral results in treating animals infected with foot and
mouth disease (results published at Congresso della
Scienze Veterinarie de Mantova, September 1970).

Fusillo states: 'Emetine hydrochloride differs from penicillin and other antibiotics because these act on bacteria
already formed, but emetine hydrochloride merely stops
viruses from proliferating, thus achieving the same thing in
a different way. Another important factor is that it stops the
viral population from taking over, without stopping the
production of antibodies which are needed to help the body
fight against the illness.'

He continues: 'There is no virus that will resist ten doses of emetine hydrochloride, there are no known side-effects and no relapses have been noted . . . The dose given is so minute that one can explain it only by hypothesizing that this poisonous vegetable extract must be a natural biological antagonist to any type of virus.'

As well as the rapid effect in herpes zoster, Fusillo comments on *the disappearance of the characteristic headache of mononucleosis*. This, too, goes within two to three days when emetine hydrochloride is used. Positive tests for mononucleosis become negative within a few weeks of emetine's employment, he claims. Since ME is thought by some doctors to be chronic mononucleosis this line of treatment should be explored.

The headache of meningo-encephalitis has also been found to disappear within 24 hours of emetine's first use. Fusillo claims equal success with other viral conditions including viral pancreatitis and viral hepatitis (A, B and C). The pain in the liver region, noted with this liver infection, is stated to disappear within a few hours of the first injection.

The medication thus appears to stop viral replication of whatever type. Ten days of therapy, Dr Fusillo states, are sufficient to deal with any viral condition.

Emetine is one of two principal constituents of ipecac, a derivative of the rhizomes of *Cephaelis ipecacuanha* or *acuminata*, which are native to Brazil and Central America. Emetine is also prepared synthetically. In doses used in the treatment of amoebic dysentery (30 to 60 milligrams injected under the skin) emetine is very irritating and its oral use is impossible due to the effects on the mucous lining of the gastro-intestinal tract. *None of these side-effects occur in the minute amounts used by Dr Fusillo, namely 2 to 3 milligrams.*

Dr Fusillo has reported on the use of emetine in the following journals: *Gazetta Medica Italiana* (February 1972),

Minarva Medica (17 January 1983) and *Manuala di Terapia Medica Regionata* (ed. Professor Rasario), seventeenth edition. It might well be that in emetine, a relatively safe antiviral agent exists, and that this could prove of value in controlling a variety of persistent viral conditions such as occur in some people with ME. This would necessarily be something to discuss fully with your medical adviser. Dr Fusillo's widow can be contacted at Via Dante, 70100 Bari, Italy.

Herbal Treatment of Viral and Other Infections

There has been a resurgence of interest in herbs of late, and especially in their safe immune-enhancing potentials and their specific antibiotic and antiviral effects. Herbs produce as good antibiotic results as do most drugs of that class, with fewer or no side-effects.

Some herbs in particular are relevant to ME: echinacea (American cornflower), hydrastis canadensis (golden-seal), radix astragalis (a Chinese medicine now widely used in alternative AIDS therapy) and glycyrrhiza glabra (licorice) which has dramatic effects on viruses of the herpes group as well as having immune-enhancing effects on the thymus gland. I will briefly describe some of the qualities of each of these.

Echinacea purpurea or angustifolia. Research has shown these remarkable herbs to have ingredients (such as inulin and echinacin) which have a potentiating (enhancing) effect on a variety of aspects of the immune system. They maintain mucous membrane integrity, thus increasing the effectiveness of this defensive barrier against infection, as well as neutralizing viruses and bacteria. Herpes family viruses (Epstein-Barr etc.) in particular are prevented from proliferating by echinacea.

Patrick Donovan in *The Textbook of Natural Medicine* provides a list of immune-enhancing results when echinacea is used and these include: stimulation of interferon production; increased macrophage activity; enhanced T-lymphocyte transformation; stimulation of production of T-lymphocytes; activation of macrophages and promotion of their activity, as well as activation of aspects of immune function known as the alternate complement pathway. (References for the research on which these claims are based are found at the end of this chapter.)

Dosage recommendations are: during active infectious phase of ME – 1 to 2 grams of dried root three times daily or 1½ to 3 ml of fluid extract three times daily.

Hydrastis canadensis. The goldenseal root has been a traditional native American medicine for thousands of years. It has a soothing effect on inflamed mucous membranes especially of the respiratory, digestive and genito-urinary tracts, whether resulting from allergy or infection.

The active ingredient appears to be berberine. This is of particular importance in infections relating to Epstein-Barr virus where berberine's influence in enhancing spleen and liver function, as well as increasing macrophage activity, makes it extremely useful as an immune-system enhancer.

Berberine has a broad-spectrum antibiotic effect against bacteria, fungi and protozoa where its effectiveness is in some instances stronger than regular medical antibiotics. In particular it is effective against candida albicans.

Dosage recommendations are: during active infectious stage of ME – 0.5 to 1 gram of dried root three times daily or 1 to 2 ml of fluid extract three times daily. During chronic or recovery phase: 300 to 500 milligrams of dried root three times daily or 0.5 to 1 ml of fluid extract three times daily.

Astragalus membranaceus radix. This species of plants has a long history of use in China for increasing overall resistance, especially in diseases which are wasting or exhausting. Studies on animals and humans confirm its benefits to the immune system, especially in viral conditions such as the common cold, where Chinese studies show it to increase levels of interferon. This is thought to make it especially useful for conditions such as ME.

Dosage recommendations: during chronic or recovery stage of ME – between 5 and 10 grams, three times daily, of dried root.

Glycyrrhiza glabra. The antiviral effects of licorice are well established, especially against the herpes family of viruses where its effectiveness is proven. It has also shown itself to be a powerful antiviral agent in cases of hepatitis. It enhances production of interferon and increases macrophage activity.

The active substances in licorice include glycyrrhizic acid, which interferes with the genetic material (DNA/RNA) of many different types of virus without interfering with the ability of the cells in which these are present to replicate normally. It has been shown to inactivate irreversibly the herpes simplex virus. It also enhances thymus gland activity.

Dosage recommendation: during active infectious stage of ME – 4 grams of dried root three times daily or 4 ml of fluid extract three times daily. During chronic or recovery stage of ME – 2 grams of dried root three times daily or 2 ml of fluid extract three times daily.

Note: Not all of these herbs would be taken at the same time. Ideally during an infectious phase one or two chosen from echinacea, hydrastis or glycyrrhiza glabra would be taken. The choice would depend somewhat on the particular symptom picture. In the recovery stage astragalus and one of the others should be used. If candida is a part of the problem or if mucous membrane inflammation exists, the choice would include hydrastis. Herpes activity is vulnerable to all of these herbal extracts. Echinacea is the most widely used antibiotic herb in the USA.

This list is by no means exhaustive but represents a sound starting-point for self-medication using safe and effective traditional methods.

Vitamin C Saturation

In Chapter 10 brief mention was made of vitamin C used in large doses as part of an antiviral strategy. In such a case the nutrient is no longer being used as a food but as a medicine, for its pharmacological effect. The use of vitamin C in this way is based on the research and clinical experience of Dr Robert Cathcart of California.

Dr Cathcart, a world-renowned orthopaedic surgeon, became interested in vitamin C when he used it on himself to treat a chronic hay fever condition. Following the advice of double Nobel prizewinner Dr Linus Pauling, Cathcart found that by taking some 200 times the recommended daily amount of the vitamin (that is taking around 15 grams daily) he cured his chronic allergy.

When some time later he developed a cold, he experimented on himself and found that to control this viral infection effectively he needed vastly more than the already large amount he was taking. In fact he did not achieve the relief he sought until his intake was 50 grams of vitamin C daily. Over the years since these self-treatment experiments, Cathcart has evolved a protocol for the use of vitamin C in the treatment of viral infections ranging from hepatitis to the common cold. Of late he has been immersed in treating people with AIDS using the same approach, with remarkable results. 'I started giving massive doses of vitamin C to AIDS patients. I used it intravenously, and the effect was amazing.'

To describe how much vitamin C a person can absorb Dr

Cathcart uses the term 'bowel tolerance'. The point of maximum bowel tolerance is reached in most people when between 10 to 15 grams are taken daily in four to six divided doses.

When doses exceed bowel tolerance diarrhoea begins. Cathcart has discovered that bowel tolerance increases proportionately with the severity of the illness experienced by the patient. For example a modest infection can increase bowel tolerance (and, Cathcart assumes, the demands of the body) to as much as 100 grams per day, and some viral infections can allow up to 200 grams of vitamin C daily to be taken without any diarrhoea.

Describing this phenomenon, American nutrition researcher Gary Null states, 'Cathcart believes that tolerance increases because larger amounts of ascorbate (the chemical form of vitamin C which the body actually uses) are being drawn off to enhance the metabolic reactions that come into play when the body fights infection.'

Vitamin C appears to have its influence on viral infections in several ways. Dr Cathcart believes that the way in which our own white blood cells attempt to deal with viruses is enhanced by vitamin C, via its action as an antioxidant. As an orthopaedic surgeon he has observed vitamin C to be able to turn off what he terms the 'inflammatory cascade' which results from local free-radical activity, and thus dramatically to reduce pain and speed healing.

Similarly in treating a virus infection with vitamin C, local detoxification and free-radical activity are altered so that white blood cells can do their job of deactivating viruses. He explains that his objective is to get this antioxidant effect into tissues where infection is operating: 'It's very difficult to force enough ascorbate into the depths of tissues affected by the disease to keep the redox potential reducing. That's where most of the free radicals are being formed. It's useless taking 500 milligrams of vitamin C and saying "well that's ten times recommended daily allowance''. That is nonsense. To pull off this ascorbate trick you've got to use enormous doses.'

Cathcart goes on: 'In most people who were otherwise well and were being treated for chronic viral diseases, they would normally get diarrhoea after 10 to 20 grams split up into four to six doses in twenty-four hours. But the astonishing thing was that the same person might be able to take 30 to 60 grams with a mild cold, 100 grams with a severe cold, 150 grams with flu and sometimes in excess of 200 grams per twenty-four hours with mononucleosis or viral pneumonias.'

When the amount which can be taken orally seems inadequate for controlling severe infections (as in AIDS, which Cathcart treats in this way) intravenous supplies of vitamin C are added to the oral intake.

Exercise, Vitamin C and the ME Patient. A particular problem for people with ME is highlighted by Cathcart's comment: 'Anyone taking the massive amounts of vitamin C should exercise since this drives the vitamin C directly into tissues involved by disease and saturates them (with vitamin C) before it spills out through the kidneys.'

As I have indicated elsewhere, exercise is usually precluded in advanced ME. Cathcart thinks otherwise. He states that with a persistent viral infection such as herpes, Epstein-Barr or chronic hepatitis simply giving vitamin C is not enough. 'It looks as though the person with Epstein-Barr is so toxic that taking ascorbate by mouth to bowel tolerance does not drive the ascorbate into the body, so we recommend that people take a double or triple dose and then go out and run . . . The problem is that when you're sick the free radicals have overcome the free radical scavenging system and you feel like hell – the last thing you want to do is exercise. *But if you saturate with ascorbate, you neutralize the free radicals and you feel good. Running drives the ascorbate into the deepest, darkest recesses of the body* [my italics].'

This is a part of Dr Cathcart's approach to conditions such as ME. It should be made clear that this is not all he does. He insists on creating a healthy bowel ecology, and this means use of acidophilus in high potency form as well as dealing with candida overgrowth. He also takes account of and deals with the host of nutritional deficiencies which he inevitably finds when people have chronic ill-health of any sort. The vitamin C aspect is one of his most powerful therapeutic weapons, but it is never used in a vacuum, without a comprehensive approach to meet the patient's needs.

In the early stages of conditions such as infectious mononucleosis (glandular fever) or other flu-like conditions which may end up as ME, saturation of the body with ascorbate is highly beneficial. It is in such infections that taking vitamin C to bowel tolerance is probably a major protector against the likelihood of developing ME.

Cathcart's Protocol. The following is a summary of Dr Cathcart's vitamin C strategy. The objective is to take enough vitamin C to almost, but not quite, cause diarrhoea. The desirable intake will vary from day to day and with the severity of the condition as well as many other factors including stress and exposure to polluted atmosphere or toxicity of any sort. In infections, bowel tolerance is between 40 and 100 grams per twenty-four hours. In acute situations this may rise well above 100 grams per twenty-four hours. Small doses should be taken hourly for best results.

The type of ascorbate taken should be balanced: 75 per cent ascorbic acid buffered with calcium, magnesium and potassium ascorbate, in powder form mixed in water. A straw should be used to prevent contact with tooth enamel.

Starting with one gram per (waking) hour, build the intake up to bowel tolerance by adding several grams per day until diarrhoea is experienced. At that time reduce to the dosage level of the previous day and maintain this until symptomatic relief is experienced, or reduce further as bowel tolerance varies. Periodically test bowel tolerance by increasing intake again to see whether the body's demand for ascorbic acid has risen.

When symptomatic relief is experienced (infection halted, temperature normal, symptoms generally relieved etc.) slowly start reducing intake at the same rate at which you increased it initially, until a maintenance dose is achieved of between 2 and 10 grams daily. Again bowel tolerance will tell you when you have reached the right level. Put up with transient diarrhoea experienced during this reducing phase and do nothing to stop it such as taking any medication. A rapid stopping of a high vitamin C intake can result in a rebound effect and a swift return of infection.

This method of trying to achieve bowel tolerance of vitamin C is presented as an option not a recommendation. Ideally it should be monitored by a professional health adviser familiar with nutritional methods in the treatment of ill-health.

You have now seen a number of possible approaches to the virus/infection problems which are often associated with ME. Which, if any, of these, is best for you depends upon many variables, including your current state of health and vitality, and the degree to which viral and other infections are contributing to your condition. One or other of these methods is almost always needed where persistent viral infection is present in cases of ME. The use of adaptogens, described in Chapter 10, is always recommended to increase overall resistance.

REFERENCES

AIDS Treatment News, 'AL721: The Deadly Silence', 2 January 1987; and 'How to Make AL721', 30 January 1987. Published by and available from John James, PO Box 411256, San Francisco, California 94141.

'The AIDS Cover-up: Medical Genocide', Null, G., *Penthouse Magazine*, December 1987.

A World without AIDS, Chaitow, L., Martin, S., Thorsons, Wellingborough 1988.

'Effect of Echinacin on Phagocytosis and Natural Killer Cells', Mose, J., *Medical Welt*, vol. 34, pp. 1463–7, 1983.

'Effects of Novel Compound (AL721) on HTLV-III Infectivity in Vitro', Sarin, P., Gallo, R., *New England Journal of Medicine*, no. 313, pp. 1289–90, 1985.

How to Live Longer and Feel Younger, Pauling, L., W. H. Freeman, Oxford 1987.

'Immunostimulatory Drugs of Fungi and Higher Plants', Wagner, H., Proksh, A., *Economic and Medicinal Plant Research*, vol. 1, Academic Press, London 1985.

'Immunostimulating Polysaccharides of Higher Plants', Wagner, V., *et al.*, Arzneim-Forsch, vol. 35, pp. 1069–75, 1985.

Physiology of Membrane Fluidity, vols 1 and 2, Shinitsky, M., CRC Press, Boca Raton, Florida 1984 (explains AL721 technology).

Prospects of a New Anti-Viral Chemotherapy, Fusillo, A. (unpublished). Report by L. Chaitow published in *Townsend Letter for Doctors*, April 1988.

Textbook of Natural Medicine, Pizzorno, J., Murray, M., JBCNM, Seattle 1987.

'Vitamin C: Titrating to Bowel Tolerance', Cathcart, R., *Medical Hypothesis*, vol. 7, pp. 1359–76, 1981.

12 Additional Healing Methods for ME

Acupuncture

It has been discovered, in the treatment of AIDS, that one of the more surprising methods of helping people has been by the use of acupuncture. In New York, at the Lincoln Hospital in the Bronx, Dr Michael Smith has been using acupuncture for this purpose since 1982 with fascinating results. The clinic sees between 150 and 200 patients daily and Dr Smith states, 'Acupuncture has been perceived as beneficial for all categories of AIDS and ARC patients. We claim that acupuncture has a long-term preventative and protective value for our patients based on their seemingly low incidence of relapse and longer survival.'

If this is true for AIDS then it is doubly so for ME, where immune depression is comparatively slight.

Dr Subhuti Dharmananda of the Institute for Preventive Health Care in Portland, Oregon has described the benefits of acupuncture given to people with prodromal symptoms which sometimes lead on to AIDS. These include: persistent weight loss, loss of appetite, diarrhoea, extreme fatigue, shortness of breath, nausea, dry cough, blurred vision, persistent fevers, night sweats and swollen lymph glands.

Anyone with ME will recognize that some of these symptoms are very familiar indeed. In traditional Chinese medicine these symptoms represent, says Dr Dharmananda, 'a combination of deficiency patterns of the spleen, lung and kidneys'. Acupuncture helps both symptomatically and by enhancing immune function, something it does very efficiently according to extensive research (see References) which shows marked (up to 70 per cent) increases in levels of leucocytes and increased levels and ratios of T-cells, after acupuncture treatment.

A further benefit for people with ME is that acupuncture, when correctly applied, seems to be one of the few treatments which leaves the individual feeling both more energetic and relaxed.

Colonic Irrigation and Enema

Colonic irrigation and enemas can be used to achieve two basic results.

1 The effective cleansing of the lower bowel (if a self-applied enema is used) or of the entire colon (if a professionally applied colonic irrigation is used), allowing removal of impacted toxic material.
2 The introduction of substances which can enhance healing, including oxygen, herbal substances and friendly bacterial cultures. This is especially valuable for anyone who has active yeast overgrowth.

Excellent results are claimed for people with ME and chronic fatigue where a variety of bowel-related factors may be in need of help, including chronic constipation, bowel toxaemia, candida overgrowth and the presence of parasites.

Colonic irrigation is not something which replaces efforts to normalize the system via nutritional and other therapeutic efforts. It is, however, a valuable additional method which in some instances has remarkably swift results. A well-qualified technician is essential, and I have provided addresses (see Resources) which will help in locating someone who fits this need.

Self-administered enemas can also be useful, especially when these are used to repopulate the bowel with acidophilus cultures or where coffee is used as a means of stimulating liver detoxification. Other agents which can be self-administered in enemas are aloe vera juice and lemon juice.

Basic enema instructions. In order to eliminate toxic debris from the lower bowel a plain water enema is used. This requires the purchasing of a syringe or gravity bag from a pharmacist. If a syringe is used, water at body heat is inserted slowly from this into the rectum while you lie on your right side, knees bent, with a thick towel under you to absorb any fluid which leaks. The end of the syringe should have been lubricated with a suitable gel. This water is retained for 5 to 15 minutes before being voided into the toilet.

If a gravity bag is used, this is suspended some two feet above your body level so that the water, at body heat, drains down an applicator tube into the lower bowel, the end of the tube having first been lubricated. Such tubes have clips which allow for the water flow to be stopped should mild discomfort be felt as the water passes into the lower colon. After a moment or two this usually ceases and the water can again be allowed to flow. After a suitable period of retention this is voided.

It is usual to suggest that during the period of retention you turn on to your left side for a few minutes, before turning on to your back and then again on to your right side. It is also often useful to gently knead the lower abdomen with your hands whilst in these positions.

The following substances can be added:

1   The addition of aloe vera juice (a teaspoonful of aloe
    vera juice per pint of water) is soothing and anti-
    fungal.
2   A teaspoonful of powdered acidophilus culture added
    to the water is another useful antifungal approach.
    This should be retained for at least 15 minutes to
    allow absorption of the acidophilus. Repopulation of
    the bowel in this way as well as by taking acidophilus
    orally is strongly advised after antibiotic therapy or if
    candida is active. If you are milk-sensitive there are
    dairy-free acidophilus cultures available. (See
    Resources section for suppliers.)
3   Far and away the finest detoxification enema is the
    plain coffee enema, devised by Dr Max Gerson in the
    1930s in treating a range of degenerative diseases, and
    still used extensively in the clinic which his daughter
    runs in North America. This is of immediate value for
    anyone feeling sensations of nausea, or who has liver
    problems. Coffee taken in enema form is transported
    directly to the liver where it stimulates the release of
    bile as well as having strong effects on peristaltic
    activity in the intestines. It is frequently found to give
    relief from headaches and nausea in a matter of
    minutes due to this release from the liver of bile which
    carries with it toxic residues.

    To make a coffee enema, add three tablespoons of
    ground coffee to two pints of water. Boil for 3 minutes
    and then allow to stand for 15 minutes. Strain this liquid
    and use one quarter of it (half-pint) at body heat for an
    enema. Store the rest in the refrigerator and warm
    before using in the same way on another occasion.

    Take this half-pint in an enema as described above
    (lying on right side etc.) and retain for a full 10
    minutes. This is not meant to cleanse the lower bowel
    but to stimulate detoxification of the liver. It can be

used as often as you wish, daily if desired, since the feeling of renewed energy and clearer head will be most welcome to many with ME and no side-effects or reactions are usual.

4 A variety of additions to enema liquid can be employed including camomile and fennel. Advice from a herbalist or therapist who uses such substances in colonic irrigations is suggested.

For names of therapists who use these methods in high colonics (the enema travels only a short distance, a colonic can traverse the entire colon) contact the Colonics International Association or the Colonic Hydrotherapy Foundation (see Resources list) and ask for the name of their nearest member to your home.

Detoxification Diets and Fasting

The simple act of stopping the eating of solid food has a rapid and beneficial short-term effect on the immune system. A report in the *Journal of the American Medical Association* in 1983 confirmed what had long been observed by naturopaths, who regularly introduce fasting in cases of acute infection.

During the initial thirty-six hours of a fast (water only) there is: increased macrophage activity; enhanced cell-mediated immune function; increased immunoglobulin levels; heightened monocyte killing activity and bactericidal activity; enhanced natural killer-cell activity; and a number of other valuable changes.

These alterations are evidence of the mobilization of the vast resources of individual aspects of the immune system in response to fasting, which acting in concert can be dramatically effective in increasing the body's defensive efficiency.

If fasting continues for longer than this short period other changes occur, some very useful in terms of overall detoxification, but there is also a reduction in immune efficiency in terms of defence against infection.

It is therefore of value for *anyone who is not severely malnourished* to stop eating for up to *but no more than*, 24 to 36 hours when any active bacterial or viral infection is current. Resistance to infection has been observed to be increased during the immediate post-fast period, which is valuable for anyone with continuing low-grade infection (virus or fungus etc.).

It should be obvious, however, that fasting should not be undertaken if there is any suggestion of malnutrition, nor – because fasting is useful sometimes – should it be undertaken too frequently (probably not more than once in six weeks unless a professional health adviser has suggested it).

The use of fasting in situations other than infection is also of value, especially as a means of improving detoxification of the system accompanied by regeneration and more speedy healing. If general nutrition is reasonable a short (48 hour) unsupervised fast can be undertaken every six weeks or so. Longer fasts must be under supervision, in a health hydro or at home with a practitioner monitoring the situation.

Ideally advice, general guidance, and possibly supervision, should be sought from a practitioner familiar with fasting, such as a clinical ecologist (a doctor specializing in allergies who uses nutritional methods including fasting) or a naturopathic practitioner. Naturopaths traditionally use fasting as a major part of their therapeutic effort and understand the many variations possible, and the way to handle the rare and unlikely, but nevertheless possible, reactions to fasting which can occur. A short fast (24–36 hours) should be introduced as early in an infection as possible.

Fasting Methods

1   During a fast eat nothing, but consume not less than 4 pints (or more than 8 pints) of water or diluted fruit juice or vegetable broth. Liquids should be consumed at two-hourly intervals or whenever desired.

2   Have a warm water enema on each day of the fast *or* three times a day drink a dose of a tablespoonful of powdered psyllium seeds (not husks or psyllium seed capsules) blended in 8 fluid ounces of spring water. Either of these methods ensures that bowel function remains operative during the fast.

3   During the fast rest as much as possible, although bed-rest is not necessary. Undertake no physical exertion and do not drive a car as a feeling of lightheadedness is common. Get some fresh air and walk a little if you are not feeling too under the weather. There may be slight feelings of nausea and/ or a headache. This is evidence of the beginning of detoxification and nothing should be done to suppress this process via medication, although a coffee enema can usually clear these symptoms rapidly.

4   Do not smoke, and stop the intake of all nutrient supplements apart from acidophilus cultures.

The fast is broken with a very light snack such as natural yogurt, a baked apple, stewed pears, or vegetable soup. Some hours later a boiled egg or steamed fish may be eaten and thereafter normal meals may be resumed. The quantity you want to eat may be reduced for some days, although appetite should be good.

To summarize, then, take a short fast if infection is current, but restrict this to 36 hours before breaking it. Take a regular 48 hour detoxification fast every six weeks, if there is no current infection and you are not physically malnourished, or seek professional supervision if a longer fast is considered.

Anyone with allergies or sensitivities may find that symptoms vanish on a fast, indeed a five-day fast is employed by many doctors seeking to unmask hidden allergies. You should be aware, though, that reactions to foods or substances may be dramatically more violent after such a fast, which is one reason for the suggestion that professional guidance be sought for any fast which is intended to last more than 48 hours.

Short fasts of the kind advocated here are never likely to present any problems, either during or afterwards.

Homoeopathic Medicine

A number of medical doctors who utilize homoeopathic medication (minute doses of medicines which in large doses would produce symptoms similar to those from which the patient is suffering) are treating ME with claimed success.

In the majority of cases reported by one such practitioner, Andrew Lockie, there was evidence of strong emotional and stress elements in the six months before the onset of the syndrome. Results of a survey showed that 70 per cent of ME patients were helped by homoeopathic medication (45 per cent were helped also by nutritional methods including supplementation).

The medication used is different in each case, since the doctor matches all the signs, symptoms and characteristics of the patient to the 'remedy'. The survey shows fully 14 different remedies to have been used successfully in dealing with ME. The fact that the remedy is aimed at the patient's characteristics rather than at the 'disease' is compatible with a holistic approach.

Homoeopathic practitioners can be found by contacting the addresses given in the Resources section.

General Life-Style Pointers

In Chapter 8 we discussed sleep, exercise and other elements involving your personal environment. The guidelines given in that chapter should be remembered especially in relation to adequate sleep, general stretching and mobilizing exercises, and the avoidance of polluted and undesirable conditions which fail to provide adequate humidity, air movement, full-spectrum light and negative ionization.

It should be absolutely clear by now that in order to provide the body with the chance of recovery, the ideal would be to ensure optimum dietary patterns with supplementation of those nutrients indicated by the condition; stress-reduction methods including physical stretching and overall lowering of arousal through relaxation techniques and improved breathing function; use, as appropriate, of antiviral and antifungal methods; all the while maintaining a certainty that recovery is not only possible but probable.

Only by a co-ordinated, holistic, rational approach can the healing of ME take place.

Can Orthodox Medical Methods Assist in Healing?

Of course they can, if they are supportive of the body's homoeostatic, self-healing efforts. But not if they are immune-suppressing or are only aimed at symptomatic relief.

The rising tide of immune-system dysfunction is evidenced by the dramatic increase in childhood allergies over the past forty years, the increase in chronic auto-immune diseases and the emergence of AIDS and of ME as major health problems in this last part of the twentieth century. All of these indicate that a shift in emphasis is required, away from the old approach of treating individual symptoms and syndromes as though they were unconnected with the total environment of the person who is suffering.

It is only by using a comprehensive approach which enhances the innate healing potentials of the body that anything like healing has taken place in some people with AIDS. The histories of the long-term survivors of AIDS are inspirational. Without exception they have reformed their dietary patterns, taken vast amounts of nutrient supplements, and used stress-reduction and relaxation/meditation/visualization methods to enhance immune function, and in most cases they have incorporated alongside aspects of orthodox methods such alternative therapies as acupuncture and herbal medicine.

Since AIDS represents the ultimate immune-system breakdown and ME could in some ways be seen as a mini-version of the same thing, the successful holistic example which these long-term survivors have given us should act as a beacon and an inspiration for people with ME.

REFERENCES

Acupuncture Treatment of AIDS, Smith, M., Rabinowitz, N., Acupuncture Clinic, Lincoln Hospital, Bronx, NY.

A Cancer Therapy: Results of Fifty Cases, Gerson, M., Totality Books, 1977.

A World Without AIDS, Chaitow, L., Martin, S., Thorsons, Wellingborough 1988.

'Colonic Cleansing', Dawson, D., *Journal of Alternative and Complementary Medicine*, pp. 31–3, May 1988.

'Fasting Enhanced Immune Effector Mechanism', Wing, E., *et al.*, *American Journal of Medicine*, vol. 75, pp. 91–6, 1983.

'Neurohumoural Modification after Acupuncture', Cracium, T., *et al.*, *American Journal of Acupuncture*, vol. 21, pp. 67–70, 1973.

Oriental Healing Arts International Bulletin, Dharmananda, S., vol. 12, no. 1, pp. 24–38, 1987.

'Preliminary Observations on the Effects of Acupuncture on Immune Response', Chy Yangming *et al.*, *American Journal of Chinese Medicine*, vol. 3, no. 2, pp. 151–63, 1975.

PVFS Survey, Lockie, A., unpublished statistics given at BRICCAP Conference, Hammersmith, London, May 1988.

'Therapeutic Fasting', Salloum, T., Burton, A., 'Fasting' in *Textbook of Natural Medicine*, Pizzorno, J., Murray, M., JBCNM, Seattle 1987.

13 Current Medical Thinking and ME

There is no consensus in the medical world as to the cause(s) of ME. A variety of tests and studies have variously blamed viral infection, food and substance allergy and sensitivity, toxicity and deficiency conditions, psychological dysfunction, congenital or acquired immune dysfunction, and hyperventilation. Even the purported viral agent(s) remain a subject for controversy.

This seems to lead to the logical conclusion, since all these researchers and practitioners are of the highest probity, that the condition is multifactorial, with many possible interacting causes; and that the ideal for recovery depends upon identification of such causes where this is possible, and the removal of these, coupled with enhancement of overall powers of self-healing through improved immune function and general health.

What is medical science currently offering the person with ME? This very much depends upon who you ask.

Allergy and Hyperventilation: Is the Mind the Link?

Many doctors are concentrating their efforts on the fact that many (some say all) people with ME have single or multiple allergies or sensitivities. Their efforts to find such allergies may be rewarded, and the approach then is to use either rotation dietary patterns to minimize exposure to particular food families, or desensitization methods which reduce or eliminate the reaction of the body to the allergen. This approach begs the question as to *why* the person first became sensitized to this food? The answer may lie in previous viral infection.

Dr Jonathan Brostoff was quoted earlier as stating: 'A particular virus may (in childhood) alter the immune function for many years, by altering the antibody levels or particular antibodies. There is no doubt in my clinic that virus infections may bring on, expose, produce or allow to be seen, an ordinary inhalant allergy (and I use allergy in the true sense, e.g. grass, pollen, house dust etc. as an ordinary type of allergy) . . . It may not have caused it, but the equilibrium may have been moved and the immunity may have become more allergy prone.' Removal of the allergic load, by desensitization or avoidance, improves the person's state of health enormously and often allows the innate self-healing capabilities of the body to then restore normality.

This works in some, but not all, patients with ME. But are allergies real or are they 'all in the mind'? Other medical researchers adopt an entirely different view. Dr Richard Cottrell, science director of the British Nutrition Foundation, says that people often react to food allergens only if they know they are in the food, and do not react if they believe that they are consuming something else: 'Genuine reactions (to food allergens) include numbness, weakness, headaches and diarrhoea, and these are common, *but only when the people tested know what they are getting.* Specialists at two or three London hospitals said they get nine patients reacting in that way to every one who reacted "blind", not knowing what the substance (which they are eating) is.'

He believes therefore that allergy is usually psychogenic, a very real response which is generated by either anxiety or the expectation of an allergic reaction. It is his view that a likely mechanism for this is hyperventilation – occurring for whatever reason – which produces a rise in blood oxygen, a disruption of the digestive process, various biochemical changes in the body, and the increased likelihood of allergy. His answer is the same as that of Dr Brostoff, avoidance of the food(s) which trigger the allergy.

This hypothesis, that many people only produce an allergic reaction to foods if they know that they are eating these foods, was shown to be more than mere conjecture by the results obtained by Dr Elspeth Young, a dermatologist at High Wycomb general hospital in Buckinghamshire who tested people with food allergies by giving them the genuine article (chocolate, milk, eggs, fish, nuts, wheat, soya etc.) as well as by supplying artificial foods made to seem just like the real thing. All the foods used in the testing were made up into bars or cans so that they appeared to be identical.

Research at Guy's Hospital, London also links hyper-ventilation and allergy, in this case asthma. Dr Tak Lee, who is professor of allergy at the hospital, has examined the inflammatory chemicals which are produced during an asthmatic attack. He says, 'We have been able to show that cells in a lung can be made to secrete these chemicals in all sorts of ways, *not only by being exposed to allergy-causing substances like pollens.'*

Another process which can have this same result, he maintains, is hyperventilaton brought on by anxiety. This can provoke the secretion of the same chemicals as the allergen. Hyperventilation can also lead to spasms of blood vessels due to the increased alkalinity of the blood caused by overbreathing. These spasms can affect the brain, the heart, and probably the lungs as well.

Dr Lee believes that, 'It is possible that both psychological and physical stimuli work through a common pathway.' For the person with ME who has to live with food and other allergies the implications are clear. Not only must the allergic element be dealt with but also the possible psychological/anxiety-related elements as well.

We are back again to the essential point that we must recognize the multifactorial, interrelating elements which allow ME (and allergy and hyperventilation and immune deficiency etc.) to occur. An attempt, say, to deal with ME by use of induced sleep and breathing retraining is no more one-sided (although it is) than is an approach which simply desensitizes the person against the allergen. No single approach can deal with the whole cause, only with part of the picture.

What about the Virus?

There are many doctors who approach the problem of ME by trying to reduce the presence or activity of ongoing infection in those cases where it can be established that this is not in fact postviral fatigue but rather persistent viral fatigue. (Perhaps persistent viral fatigue syndrome should be yet another name to add to the many which this condition has already acquired.)

Dr David Smith tells us, 'In the group of people I have studied and who I believe have postviral syndrome clinically, if you look for evidence of old Coxsackie virus infection, then you will find 35 per cent of these people have very significantly raised antibody titres (high levels of Coxsackie-B virus immunoglobulin G). It indicates that they have had virus infection in the past. If you look at lower levels of antibodies you find that 70 per cent of this group of people show evidence of old Coxsackie infection. In the normal population the incidence is 5 per cent. This is significant but it proves nothing [i.e. it does not actually provide evidence of causation].'

'If you look for evidence of ongoing Coxsackie infection by looking for immunoglobulin M, 17 per cent of the study group have strongly positive evidence for current Coxsackie virus infection. In the normal population this would be 0.5 per cent. In other words it is 34 times more significant than normal. Again it proves nothing.'

Dr Smith uses gamma globulin (IgG) injections to enhance immune function in such cases. This is the antibody which people make in response to various antigens. He explains its source: 'If you take blood plasma from the blood products laboratory after it has been deemed no longer of use for transfusion (approximately a month after donation) you can take away all the red cells, all the white cells and all the other bits and pieces and you can concentrate the various people's antibodies and that is what gamma globulin is.'

He has used gamma globulin in appropriate cases (750 milligrams each month intramuscularly) and claims that two-thirds of the patients receiving this have significantly improved. He acknowledges that this benefit may be a placebo effect (in which whatever is done to a group of patients, valid or not, some will improve). He also acknowledges: 'We may [by using gamma globulin] be helping your own immune system in a logical way to fight that particular infection that you cannot fight appropriately. Gamma globulin is a passive vaccination. It just mops up the antigen in your blood. *It does not do very much in the way of stimulating your immune system.*'

The recently reported finding by Professor Mowbray, in

The Lancet (23 January 1988), which showed that a significant number of people with ME have persistent, chronic,
enterovirus (Coxsackie-B and others) infection in their
bowels should indicate that at least in such people short-
term use of gamma globulin is likely to solve little, because
the reservoir of viral activity would remain in the bowel,
constantly and persistently reinfecting the system whenever immune function was weak.

It is not until the bowel immune function is adequate to
dealing with these interlopers that health will be restored in
such cases. Again an holistic approach which deals with
bowel health and general health is called for. Dr A. Melvyn
Ramsey of the Royal Free Hospital, London, stated in
relation to ME in 1981, 'The particular invading microbial
agent is probably not the most important factor. Recent
work suggests that the key to the problem is likely to be
found in the abnormal immunological response of the
patient to the organism.'

The Susceptibility Element

Here we come close to the heart of the matter. Dr Patrick
Donovan has suggested that the approach which tries to
focus on the virus is doomed to failure: 'Susceptibility is the
state of being easily influenced by or affected with disease.
The importance of susceptibility is overlooked in the
disease/infection equation which continues to dominate
[allopathic] medicine. This neglect is readily apparent in the
current treatment approaches found in medical diagnostic
texts, which focus almost completely on the reduction or
elimination of the supposedly causative agent or the control
of a symptom or manifestation of a disease process (the
tumour, the headache etc.). Little attention is paid to the
host's susceptibility. . . . The key to cure lies in the
reduction and elimination of susceptibility and this should

be the primary focus of therapy. Susceptibility to infection and disease can be reduced and eliminated only by building optimal health and integrity of the total organism. *All aspects and levels of function, from the spiritual and psycho-emotional to the biochemical, must be addressed. At the centre is the immune system. It is the fulcrum or key point upon which health and disease, resistance and susceptibility, are balanced* [my italics].'

It is my contention that here lies the road to recovery – in paying attention to the total needs of the body and mind (and spirit) and in avoiding the use of short-term answers for anything but short-term needs.

Nowhere is this more clearly demonstrated than in the use of antifungal drugs in treating candida albicans. Nystatin is the standard medical answer to candida overgrowth. It does kill yeast very effectively, but does nothing whatever to enhance the natural control of this lifelong inhabitant of our body, which having been impaired by antibiotics, steroids (contraceptive pill etc.) and a high sugar content in the diet, cannot be regained simply by killing the yeast. Restoration of control requires repopulation of the bowel with natural flora and this needs to be combined with antifungal tactics which do not produce a rebound of candida when they cease, such as often occurs when nystatin is abruptly stopped.

Nothing but an holistic approach, which aims at restoring to the body its prerogative and ability for healing itself, will adequately deal with candida, or ME, or any other illness.

An antiviral, anti-candida, immune-enhancing, energy-promoting, stress-reducing, function-improving approach is called for if we are to deal with anything other than just one aspect of the problem which is ME. This calls for the patient to accept most of the responsibility for recovery.

188

It is my hope that the information provided in this book will help you to accept the challenge, and to meet it.

REFERENCES

'Chronic Enterovirus Infection in Patients with PVFS', Yousef, G., Mowbray, J., *et al.*, *The Lancet*, 23 January 1988, pp. 146–9.

'Chronic Mononucleosis-Like Syndrome', Donovan, P., Chapter 6 in *Textbook of Natural Medicine*, Pizzorno, J., Murray, M., JBCNM, Seattle 1987.

'Imaginary Allergies the Key to Real Ills', Hodgkinson, N., *Sunday Times*, 3 July 1988, p. A3.

Internal Medicine, ed. Stein, J., Little, Brown, Boston 1983.

'Medical Addresses Given at 1985 AGM of UK ME Association', report in Journal of the ANZ ME Society, May 1986.

Myalgic Encephalomyelitis: A Baffling Syndrome, Ramsay, A. M., published by ME Association, November 1981.

List of Resources

Suppliers

Amino acids, vitamins, minerals, raw glandular extracts etc. can be obtained by post from:

Cantassium Co., 225 Putney Bridge Road, London SW15 2PY (01-874-1130)

G&G Supplies, 175 London Road, East Grinstead, Sussex (0342-23016)

Nature's Best, PO Box 1, Tunbridge Wells, Kent (0892-34143)

Natural Flow, Burwash Common, East Sussex (0435-882482)

Yeast-free B vitamins are available by post from:
Bio-Health, 13 Oakdale Road, London SW16 (01-769-7975)

Capricin (anti-fungal coconut extract) and high-potency enzyme supplements are available by post from:
BioCare, 20–24 High Street, Solihull, West Midlands B91 3TB (021-705-4975)

High potency acidophilus (Superdophilus brand recommended) and other lactobacilli, including milk-free varieties, are available by post from:

G&G Supplies, 175 London Road, East Grinstead, Sussex (0342-23016)

For probion (bowel flora bacterial culture) supplement and organic germanium contact:
Symbiogenesis, BCM Box 22, London WC1 3XX

Adaptogens and herbal products are available by post from:
Salus-Haus, Fern Reach, Delph Lane, Daresbury, Warrington, Cheshire (0925-74326)

Herbal supplies available by post from:
Neals Yard Apothecary, 2 Neals Yard, London WC2 *or*
Potters Herbal Supplies, Leyland Mill Lane, Wigan, Lancashire (0942-34761)

Ionizers and air-purifying equipment available from:
The Novo Centre, 9–11 London Lane, London E8 3PR (01-986-4717)
Oasis, 50 Esplanade, Poole, Dorset BH15 2BA (0202-672423)
Selectair Ltd, Beckett's Wharf, Lower Teddington Road, Hampton Wick, Kingston-on-Thames (01-943-4144)

VM1 the AL721 'clone' is available by contacting 01-299-1409

Practitioners/Specialist Help

Hair mineral analysis for toxic heavy metals:
BioMed International, 55 Queens Road, East Grinstead, Sussex RH19 1BG (0342-22854). Cost is under £20
New Era Laboratory, Marfleet, Hull HU9 1BR (0482-75234). Cost is under £20

Nutritional analysis and advice are available from:
Green Farm Nutrition Centre, Burwash, East Sussex TN19 7LX (0435-882180)
Institute for Optimum Nutrition, 5 Jerdan Place, Fulham, London SW6 1BE (01-485-7984)

Resources

Medabolics, Broadway House, 14 Mount Pleasant Road, Tunbridge Wells, Kent TN1 1QU (0892-42609)

Acupuncture practitioners. Contact:
British Acupuncture Association and Register, 34 Alderny Street, London SW1V 4EU (01-834-1012)

Allergy specialists (clinical ecologists and those involved in environmental medicine). Contact:
Action Against Allergy, 43 The Downs, London SW20 8HG (01-947-5082) *or*
British Society of Allergy and Environmental Medicine, Burghwood Clinic, 34 Brighton Road, Banstead, Surrey SM17 1BS (07373-61177). (Medical practitioners only) *or*
British Society for Clinical Ecology, Royal Liverpool Hospital, Liverpool L7 9XP (051-709-0141). (Medical practitioners only) *or*
The Environmental Medicine Foundation, c/o Montrose, 111 Toms Lane, Kings Langley, Herts WD4 8NP

Autogenic training. Contact:
Dr Kai Kermani, 10 Connaught Hill, Loughton, Essex 1G10 4DU. (*Note* Dr Kermani specializes in helping people with AIDS with autogenic training. He can refer you to teachers with a wider range of therapeutic interest.)

Chelation therapy. Contact:
Centre for Chelation Therapy, 3 The Glade, Pagham, West Sussex (0243-263624)

Colonic irrigation therapists. Contact:
Colonics International Association, 26 Sea Road, Boscombe, Bournemouth, Dorset BH5 1DF *or*
Colonic Hydrotherapy Foundation, 62 Alexandra Road, Hemel Hempstead, Herts

Dental practitioners who specialize in amalgam replacement.
Contact:
Dental Society for Clinical Nutrition, c/o 1 Welbeck House,
62 Welbeck Street, London W1M 7HB (01-486-3127) *or*
Glenrose, Bernards Close, Great Missenden, Bucks (02406-
4601/5997)

Medical practitioners who use holistic or nutritional methods.
Contact:
British Holistic Medical Association, 179 Gloucester Place,
London NW1 6DX (01-262-5299)
British Society for Nutritional Medicine, PO Box 3AP,
London W1A 3AP

Homoeopathic practitioners. Contact:
British Homoeopathic Association, 27a Devonshire Street,
London W1N 1RJ (01-935-2163). (Medical practitioners
only)
The Faculty of Homoeopathy, The Royal London Homoeo-
pathic Hospital, Great Ormond Street, London WC1N 3HR
(01-837-8833 ext. 72 or 85). (Medical practitioners only)
Register and Council of Homoeopathy, 243 The Broadway,
Southall, Middlesex (01-574-4281). (Lay homoeopathic
practitioners)

Naturopathic practitioners (specializing in nutrition and fasting).
Contact:
BNA, 6 Netherhall Gardens, London NW3 5RR (01-435-
8728) and ask for national list of qualified practitioners

Osteopathic practitioners. Contact:
General Council and Register of Osteopaths, 1–4 Suffolk
Street, London SW1 4HG (01-839-2060) and ask for national
list of qualified practitioners

Yoga teachers specializing in helping the disabled and those with specific health problems. Contact:
Yoga for Health Foundation, Ickwell Bury, Nr Biggleswade, Bedfordshire (Northill 271)

Myalgic Encephalomyelitis Support Groups

The ME Action Campaign, PO Box 1126, London W3 0RY
The ME Association, PO Box 8, Stanford le Hope, Essex
The Australian and New Zealand ME Society, PO Box 47–191, Ponsonby, Auckland 1, New Zealand
CFSS (Chronic Fatigue Syndrome Society), PO Box 230108, Portland, Oregon 97223, USA.

Index

acidophilus 25, 59, 61, 64, 66, 121–2, 168,
174, 177
acne 70
acupuncture 144, 171–2
adaptogens 126–7, 169
Ader, Dr Robert 37–8
adrenal exhaustion 86, 90
adrenalin 86
aerobic exercise 92
AIDS 23–6, 55–6, 150–2, 155–9, 165, 167,
171, 179–80
holistic treatment of vii, 136, 148, 180
air-conditioning 95
alcohol 56, 86, 90, 104, 105
allergies 7, 13, 33, 37, 40, 47, 49, 62, 63, 70,
72, 85, 87, 89–90, 101, 117–18, 129,
151, 179–80
and breast feeding 54
environmental 12, 55, 95–7
and fasting 178
and immunization/
vaccination 55
and ME 47, 52–9, 68, 183–5
and stress 35, 58
aloe vera 123, 173–4
AL721 28, 155–9
alternative medicine vii, 171–80
amino acids 51, 81, 103, 106, 113–17, 154
arginine 79, 113–17, 124, 154–5
carnitine 82, 117, 125
cysteine 51, 126
L-glutamine 124
lysine 79, 113–17, 124, 154–5

methionine 51, 126
tryptophan 94, 119
anaemia 50
anorexia 50
antibiotics 53–4, 62–3, 67–8, 90, 103, 105,
174, 188
antioxidants 119, 166
anxiety vii, 44–5, 49, 86, 129, 184
attacks 6, 7, 42
appetite, loss of 7, 171
arousal, reducing 129, 144–52, 179
arthritis 21, 37, 50, 84
ascorbate 166–9
asthma 49, 53–5, 56, 184
astralagus 162, 163–4
ataxia 42
athlete's foot 70
autogenic training (A.T.) 136–40, 147–8,
150
AZT 26

bacterial infections 11, 25, 53–4, 62–3, 90
see also fungal; viral
Baldwin, Jay 150
B-cells 34, 80
Beard, Dr 3, 32
behaviour patterns, changing 132–5
bifido factor 122–3
biofeedback 40
bioflavonoids 117
Blanco-Dalmau, Professor 50
Bland, Professor Jeffrey 90

Index

blood sugar levels 56, 63, 79, 82, 85–8, 90, 102, 104, 188
bowel
   problems 172–5, 187
   tolerance to vitamin C 121, 166–9
breathing
   difficulties 42–6, 50, 171
   retraining vii, 44–6, 130, 136, 144–7, 179
   see also hyperventilation; yoga
Brostoff, Dr Jonathan 53–4, 66, 183, 184
burn-out vii, 32, 91, 93
Buttram, Dr Harold 55

calcium 51, 73, 94, 104, 120, 122
cancer 25, 37, 84, 148, 149–50, 152, 155
candida albicans
   and allergies 68–9
   and antibiotics 53–4, 67, 69–70, 90
   and diet/supplements 64, 66, 72, 78, 81–2, 101–4, 111, 118–19, 121–3
   and ME 54, 61–71
   overgrowth vi, vii, 11, 16, 24, 40, 46, 47, 54, 61–71, 97, 129, 151, 163, 168, 172, 174, 188
   symptoms 63, 70–1
Cappo, Bruce 145
caprylic acid 66, 122
Cathcart, Dr Robert 165–9
central heating 95–6, 97
cereals 54, 105, 107–8, 115
chelation, oral/intravenous 59, 125–6
Cheraskin, Professor Emanuel 75, 80
chiropractic treatment 46, 136, 144
chromium 75, 79, 88, 102, 125
chronic
   Epstein-Barr virus syndrome 4, 16, 23, 75
   fatigue syndrome (CFS) 4
   mononucleosis-like syndrome 4, 18, 161
   see also ME
circulation 84, 137
closet AIDS 4, 5
coenzyme-Q$_{10}$ 79, 83, 124
coffee, as an enema 174–5
cold
   common 164, 165–7
   sores 17
colitis 37, 49
colonic irrigation 57, 172–5
concentration, lack of 5, 7, 20
constipation 70, 172
'coping skills' 12, 16, 34–7, 89, 129, 130–2
cortisone 62, 70
Cottrell, Dr Richard 183

cough, persistent 7, 171
Coxsackie-B virus 8, 15, 17, 19–21, 23, 26, 80, 185
cystitis 70
cytomegalovirus 8, 15, 16, 19, 24, 62, 112, 156, 158

dairy produce 106, 111, 114–15
   see also milk
Davies, Stephen 58
Dawes, Dr Belinda 16, 69
deficiencies vi, 75, 80–8, 90, 93
   see also nutrition; supplements
depression vi, vii, 6, 7, 19, 23, 24, 49, 56, 63, 70, 91, 134
   and ME 10, 34
desensitization 54, 183
detoxification 102, 175–6
Dharmananda, Dr Subhuti 171
diabetic state 62, 85
diarrhoea 70, 166–7, 171
diet 101–19
   and nutritional needs 74–88, 179
   rotation/exclusion 57, 103, 183
   unbalanced 23
digestion
   aids to 83, 102–3, 109, 118–19, 121–3
   complaints 63, 70, 103, 129
dizziness 6, 42, 56
Donovan, Dr Patrick 6, 21, 23–4, 56, 75, 163, 187
drugs
   allergies 7
   side-effects 26
   sleeping 93–4
   see also antibiotics
Duesberg, Professor Peter 24

echinacea 162–3
eczema 49, 50, 53–5
eggs 54, 108, 115
emetine hydrochloride 159–62
emotional problems 20, 31, 50
   and viruses 23–4
endometriosis 70
enemas 172–5
energy 12, 44–5, 77–8, 83–8, 117, 123–5, 129, 135
enterovirus 8, 19, 26, 62–3, 187
   nucleic acid (RNA) 19–20, 164
environment, and ME 89–90, 95–7, 179
   see also air-conditioning; central heating; pollution; 'sick building syndrome'
enzymes, digestive 84–5, 103, 106, 119, 121

epidemic neuromyasthenia (ME) 4
Epstein-Barr virus (EBV) 7, 8, 15–18, 21–4,
    36, 62, 75, 112, 154–8, 162–3, 167
essential fatty acids 120
evening primrose oil 120
exercise 12, 91–2, 135–44, 167–8, 179
exhaustion vii, 11, 103, 124, 151
    see also fatigue

faintness 42
fasting 57, 175–8
fatigue vi, 5–7, 17, 19, 22, 24, 31, 43, 50, 56,
    63, 70, 87, 95, 123, 171
fats 82, 90
fermented food 103–5, 120
fever 5, 17, 114, 171
fibre 82
Finlay, Sue vi–viii, 63–5, 104
fish 108, 109, 114
flour 104, 105
fluid retention 56
food
    additives 105–6
    allergies vi, 7, 12, 101
    combinations 110, 116
    see also diet; nutrition
free radicals 83–5, 167
fruit 102, 105–6, 108, 111
fungal infections 25, 70, 104, 122–3
Fusillo, Dr Antonio 159–62

Gallo, Dr Robert 155
gamma globulin 186
garlic capsules 122
gastro-intestinal complaints 6, 7, 19, 56
germanium 79, 83, 122, 124
Gerson, Dr Max 174
ginseng 127
glands, swollen 6, 7, 17, 114, 171
glandular fever 7, 17–18, 36, 161, 167–8
glutamic acid 124
glycyrrhiza glabra 162, 164
Goldberg, Dr Philip 93
guided imagery 40, 130, 148–52

hair analysis 52, 59
hardiness factor 37, 39, 130–2
hay fever 7, 165
headache 5, 6, 17–19, 42, 49, 50, 56, 63,
    96–7
healing, and the mind 149–52
heart problems 42–3, 84–5
herbal remedies 28, 162–5
herpes 7, 17, 24, 79, 156, 158, 162, 164, 167

nutritional treatment of 112–18, 154–9,
    162, 164, 167
simplex 17, 24, 79, 164
zoster (shingles) 160–1
HIV 155, 157
Hodgkinson, Neville 92
Holmes, Dr David 146
    Pamela 15–16
homoeopathic remedies 31, 178
Hughson, Dr Mark 16
hydrastis 162, 163
hydrochloric acid 121
hypertension 50
hyperventilation vi, vii, 11, 16, 35, 42–6,
    129, 130, 135, 146, 147, 183–5
hypnosis 40
hypoglycaemia 12, 56, 82, 85–8, 101, 104–
    106, 112, 118, 125–6
'hysterical illnesses' 3–4, 8, 9, 32–3

Icelandic disease (ME) 3
immune system vi, vii, 62, 187–8
    and allergies/deficiencies 9, 47, 52–9,
        68, 82, 84, 185
    and antibiotics/drugs 26, 62, 68–9
    enhancement vii, 39–40, 101–2, 119–21,
        127, 130–2, 137, 154–69, 171, 175–6,
        180, 186
    and immunization/
        vaccination 55
    and metal toxicity 48–52
    and nutrition/
        supplements 72–90, 101–28
    and psychological factors 33–40, 89
    and stress 11, 33–40
    and viral activity 22–4, 27–8, 35, 53–4
immunization 55
infectious mononucleosis *see* glandular
    fever
interferon (IFN) 26–7, 163, 164
ions, negative and positive 96–7, 179
iron 80, 81

James, John 156, 158
joints, aching and painful 5, 22, 56, 70, 142

Kagan, Dr Christopher 113
Kaufman, Dr Daniel 93
Kermani, Dr Kai 136
kidney disorders 50

lactobacillus
    acidophilus 25, 59, 61, 64, 66, 121–2,
        168, 174, 177
    bulgaricus 61, 122

Index

lecithin 28, 155–9
Lee, Dr Tak 184–5
legionnaire's disease 97
lifestyle 13, 95–7, 130–52
  see also stress
light, full-spectrum 96–7, 179
liver disorders 17–18, 50, 161, 173
Lockie, Dr Andrew 7, 31, 178
low blood sugar 56, 79, 82, 85–8, 90
lymphocytes 8, 34, 80, 163

magnesium 81, 104, 120, 122
manganese 104
Manning, Betsy Russell 49
Martin, Simon 150, 156
massage 45, 136, 144
McEvedy, Dr 3, 32
ME 3–14, 27, 56
  Association 31, 67
  causes of 5, 11–12, 27, 182–8
  diet/supplements for 64, 69, 72–88,
    101–19, 119–28, 167–9
  healing of 12–14, 28–9, 91–7, 171–80,
    187–8
  psychological factors 7, 9–10, 16, 23,
    33–40, 56
  sufferers 11, 32, 93
  susceptibility factor 5, 187–8
  symptoms 5–14
meat 106–9, 114
meditation 40, 133, 147–52
memory problems 5, 49–50, 70
meningitis 19
meningo-encephalitis 161
menu suggestions 110–11
migraine 42, 54, 56
milk 54, 105, 114, 174
Minimata disease 49
mononucleosis see glandular fever
Mowbray, Professor James 52–3, 186–7
multiple sclerosis 50, 52, 53
muscular
  aches and pains 5, 6, 8, 17, 21, 50, 56, 70,
    92, 140, 143–4
  exercises 135–44
  tension 42–6, 129
myalgic encephalomyelitis (ME) 4

natural killer cell activity (NKCA) 34–5
nausea 7, 19, 42, 171
New Zealand ME Association 64, 137
Newton, Tony 157
Null, Gary 166
numbness 6, 19, 42, 49, 70
nutrition 12

antiviral 112–18, 154–9, 162, 164, 167
deficiencies vi, vii, 11, 13, 16, 40, 46, 69,
  85, 129
and the immune system 72–88
and ME 24, 28–9, 168, 178
nuts 113, 115
nystatin 64, 66–7, 188

olive oil 107, 109, 122
osteopathic treatment 45, 136, 144
over-breathing see hyperventilation
ozone layer 55

pain 5, 6, 8, 17, 21–2, 50, 56, 70, 92, 140–4,
  152
palpitations 6, 42
pancreatic problems 86–7, 90, 161
panic attacks 6, 20, 42, 44
Pauling, Dr Linus 165
Pearsall, Dr Paul 58, 81
penicillin 62
  see also antibiotics
physiotherapy 144
poliomyelitis 19
pollen extracts 127
pollution 55–6, 96–7, 168, 179
Poskanzer, Dr David 32
Post-Isometric Relaxation (PIR) 140–42
postviral fatigue syndrome (PVFS) vii, 4, 5
prostatitis 70
protein 81, 102, 109, 110, 118, 121
psychoneuroimmunology 9, 37–8, 40
psychotherapy 40, 45, 132
pulse/grain dishes 106, 109, 111–12, 114–
  115

Quesada, Professor 160

Ramsey, Dr A. Melvyn 187
rash, skin 17, 56, 97
Reciprocal Inhibition (RI) 140–2
relaxation, exercises and techniques 40,
  58–9, 92, 95, 130, 135–44, 148–52, 179
Revici, Dr Emanuel 24–6, 38, 62
Rost, Peter 157
Rowe, Chris 76
Royal Free disease vi, 3, 32
royal jelly 127
rubella 21

salads 109, 110
salt 107, 108
selenium 75, 81, 84, 105, 119
senile dementia 50
sense disturbances 6, 70

Sheldon, Dr Herbert 94
shingles 160
Shinitsky, Dr Meir 155
'sick building syndrome' 55, 95–7
siestas 93, 95
Simonton, Carl and Stephanie 148–50, 152
Skornik, Dr Yahuda 157
sleep
  disturbances 6, 7, 13, 20, 23, 43, 93
  and ME 92–5, 179
  pills 93–4
Smith
  Dr David 31, 67, 185–6
  Dr Michael 171
snacks 106, 109
soft tissue manipulation 45, 136, 143–4
Solomon, George 40
soya 110, 115
speech disturbances 50
steroids 62, 70, 90, 188
Stewart
  Alan 58
  Warren 76
stimulants, artificial 86, 87, 90, 105
stress 35, 43–6, 58, 86–8, 129, 168
  and diet/supplements 73–4, 79–80
  and the immune system 33–40
  and ME 31–40, 129–34
  reduction vii, 13, 16, 58, 59, 80, 127,
    129–52, 179
  -related illness vi, 7, 23
  see also coping skills
stretching exercises 92, 135–44, 179
sugar 63, 81–2, 85–8, 90, 102, 104, 188
supplements, importance of 51, 57, 72–4,
    78, 101–4, 117–28, 178–9
  and ME 72–88, 101–3, 119–28, 167–9
'susceptibility factor' 5, 187–8

T-cells 34, 80, 155, 172
throat, sore 6, 17, 114
thrush see candida
thymus extract 127
tobacco 13, 86, 90, 105
toxicity
  fungicides 90
  hair analysis 52, 59
  and ME 47, 48–52
  metal vi, 11, 13, 47, 50–2, 90, 126–7, 129,
    168
  pesticides 11, 90
trembling, tremors 42, 49
trigger points 140, 143–4

urticaria 49

vaccinations 8, 21, 22, 55
vaginitis 70
varicella-zoster virus 21, 112
vegetables 106, 109
viral
  hepatitis 161, 164, 165, 167
  infections vii, 4, 11, 16, 33, 40, 90, 112,
    129, 185–7
  pancreatitis 161
  pneumonia 167
viruses 15–29
  diet/supplements 78–80, 101, 112–18,
    154–69
  and ME 15–29, 33, 52–4, 62–3, 112–14,
    154–69, 185–7
  treatment 26–8, 53–4
  see also Coxackie-B; cytomegalovirus;
    enteroviruses; Epstein-Barr; herpes
visual disturbances 19, 42, 50, 71, 103, 171
visualization 40, 130, 138, 148–52
vitamin
  A 75, 80, 81, 84, 104, 119, 120
  B complex 75, 120
  B_1 (thiamin) 81, 104
  B_2 (riboflavin) 81, 104
  B_3 104
  B_5 (pantothenic acid) 57, 75, 80, 81, 104
  B_6 (pyridoxine) 75, 80, 81, 93, 94, 104,
    120
  B_{12} 75, 80
  biotin 61, 66, 108, 122
  folic acid 75, 80, 81
  C 51, 57, 73, 75, 81, 104, 117, 119, 120,
    165–9
  D 81
  E 81
VM_1 156–9
vomiting 7, 50

weight fluctuations 56, 171
Weiner, Dr Michael 81
Werbach, Professor Melvyn 81
Williams, Professor Roger 73, 124
Wood, Dr Clive 130–1
Wookey, Dr Celia 10–11, 68
'woolly brain syndrome' 5

yeast
  -based supplements 103, 120
  'burn off' 123
  overgrowth see candida
yoga 92, 136, 144–6
Young, Dr Elspeth 184
'yuppie flu' viii, 4, 9, 16

zinc 75, 80, 81, 84, 120